Reinvent Yourself with

color

me

beautiful

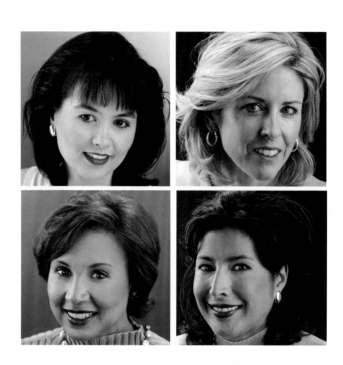

Reinvent Yourself with

color
me
beautiful

JoANNE RICHMOND

taylor trade publishing

Lanham ‖ New York ‖ Boulder ‖ Toronto ‖ Plymouth, UK

Published by Taylor Trade Publishing
An imprint of The Rowman & Littlefield Publishing Group, Inc.
4501 Forbes Boulevard, Suite 200, Lanham, Maryland 20706
www.rlpgtrade.com

Distributed by NATIONAL BOOK NETWORK

Library of Congress Cataloging-in-Publication Data

Richmond, JoAnne, 1951–
  Reinvent yourself with color me beautiful / JoAnne Richmond.
    p. cm.
  Includes index.
  ISBN-13: 978-1-58979-288-3 (pbk. : alk. paper)
  ISBN-10: 1-58979-288-2 (pbk. : alk. paper)
  1. Beauty, Personal. 2. Cosmetics. I. Title.

RA778.R483 2008
646.7'2—dc22   2007049888

∞™ The paper used in this publication meets the minimum requirements of American National Standard for Information Sciences—Permanence of Paper for Printed Library Materials, ANSI/NISO Z39.48-1992.

Manufactured in Canada.

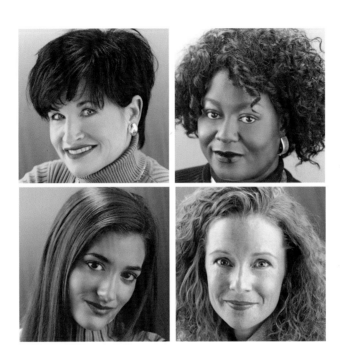

contents

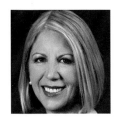

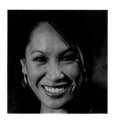

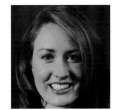

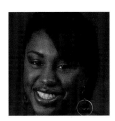

preface

I t wasn't luck that propelled the first Color Me
Beautiful book to become a major bestseller, creating
a sensation that continues to change lives today. It in-
troduced a whole new way of looking at clothes and
makeup. Like the first Color Me Beautiful book more
than a decade ago, this updated guidebook will change
your outlook on life. The concepts you'll find here will
give you the right tools to make the right choices at
home and in the store. If you haven't organized your
closet in a while or find yourself unsure about what to
buy, this is the book for you. This handy guide provides a
springboard to the concepts, colors, and regimens that
can make you look your best. Inside, you'll find great
new information and perspectives for the new millennia
. . . and a few all-new colors too.

The Color Me Beautiful concepts have been devel-
oped to give you more flexibility than ever before. We
have blended two all-new color concepts, *warm* and *cool*,
with our tried-and-true Four Seasons color palettes—
Winter, Summer, Autumn, and Spring—to help you better
understand and choose the hues for you. You'll be
stunned by the results.

Reinvent Yourself with Color Me Beautiful takes you through the Color Me Beautiful analysis just as if one of our consultants were walking you through each step to determine your best shades, best styles, and best combinations. This book's thorough analysis has been customized so that you can put it to the test at home or with friends, making it even more convenient than ever.

Do you color your hair? Well, then we've got you covered. Do you need to update your makeup? This is the place to learn how to do it. Do you need some direction when shopping through all the amazing new colors—and determine whether they are really "new"? We give you ideas on how to wear colors in ways you never have before. If that little black dress isn't a good color on you, we'll show you how to wear it to its best effect by wearing something complementary in *your* season.

As the world has become smaller, the choices have grown dramatically. Don't make the wrong one. Let Color Me Beautiful lend a hand, whether your skin tone is the deepest ebony or the palest olive. You will find our color analysis life-changing. Learn what generations of women have known about this revolutionary approach to make a change of a lifetime.

acknowledgments

This book is about my clients, the women who helped me develop an understanding of how and why the concepts of Color Me Beautiful work. Thank you to all of the women who have graced my "magic chair" and shared your insights with me. Without you this book would not have been possible.

I would also like to express a special note of appreciation to Mr. Steve DiAntonio, president and CEO of Color Me Beautiful. I want to extend my heartfelt appreciation to Lucinda Law for her vision and expertise and to Clare Sokolsky and Shirley Froemming for sharing their thoughts, knowledge, and experience. A special thank you to Mark and Rachael Palmer, my talented photographer and illustrator. The continued enthusiastic support of all of these people made this book happen.

the
first
impression

Using Color to Make Your Best Impression

Slowly count to seven: one one thousand . . . two one thousand . . . three one thousand . . . four one thousand . . . five one thousand . . . six one thousand . . . seven one thousand. That's how long it takes to form a first impression. Within seven seconds of meeting you, perfect strangers will make decisions that may have an enormous impact on your life. Are you someone they want to work with? Someone who can be trusted? Are you friend material? Should they buy your product? Color Me Beautiful wants the first impression you make to be your *best*. Help each new person to decide yes. Yes, they want to hire you! Yes, he wants to date you! Yes, she does want to get to know *you*!

In this chapter and those following it, you'll read about women like you who wanted a better understanding of how color could work for—and not against—them. Through their stories, you'll see how Color Me Beautiful's techniques that helped them can help you. With this understanding in place, you will determine your best palette, based on your hair color, skin tone, and eye color. After reading this book you will know which colors to wear, what tone of jewelry looks best on you, and which shades of lipstick, blush, and eye shadow suit you to perfection.

Let's begin with a diagnostic that will assess where you are today.

- Do you have clothing in your wardrobe that you have never worn?
- If you color your hair, do you question whether you chose the correct *warm* or *cool* tone for your hair?
- Do you receive compliments on only one or two outfits in your entire wardrobe?
- Do your clothes rarely coordinate with each other, making it impossible to streamline your wardrobe?
- Does every blush in your makeup drawer clash with the rest of your makeup, as well as each piece of clothing that you own?
- Do you have a cabinet full of makeup mistakes and wear only a few tried-and-true favored shades?
- Do you consider yourself a trend-follower rather than a trendsetter?
- Are you stuck with the same old accessories because you do not feel confident?

If you answered "yes" to one or more of these questions, there is a strong likelihood that you are making the wrong color selections. Don't worry, though! This guidebook will help you to turn the answers to these questions around.

If you follow the Color Me Beautiful color-analysis system, not only will you look years younger, but you will also spend less time shopping because you will only select the colors in your seasonal palette. Plus, you will spend less money because you will like everything that you purchase. But it doesn't have to happen overnight. Don't feel that your entire wardrobe is scheduled for the scrap heap. Ease yourself into your new world of color. This is how it happened for a few women.

Consider Jo, a classy British woman who turned her life around using the Color Me Beautiful analysis. Jo was in a funk and didn't like what she saw in the mirror. Weight gain, low self-esteem, and poor color choices had obscured to Jo what the rest of the world saw: a pretty face and a sweet smile. Color Me Beautiful showed Jo the stunning woman who was hiding under the wrong colors.

During her color analysis, Jo was wearing a fuchsia twinset and makeup that matched, which is a *cool* palette ensemble. But Jo's striking red hair, green eyes with gold flecks, and light freckled skin tone required a completely different look. By draping *warm* palette colors on her shoulders and around her face, Jo could immediately see the difference. Her eyes sparkled, and her smile appeared brighter. The fine lines around her eyes seemed to soften and diminish, and her skin tone blended with her new colors. She left that appointment a changed person. Jo started purchasing clothes in her *warm* colors. Her posture, smile, and confidence improved with the many compliments she received. A proud mother of three, when she walks into a room she glows!

The Color Me Beautiful analysis can also help you when choosing your ideal hair color. Take Eileen, a teacher. This very intelligent woman was a recent widow who was afraid of her future. In a rash act, Eileen had returned to her hair color of a happier, safer time: her twenties. It looked terrible. After Eileen looked at herself draped in her *cool* palette colors, she was easily persuaded that her recent hair color choice was too intense. Eileen looks beautiful and elegant with her corrected hair coloring and best shades of clothing and makeup. And she has started dating again!

Anne Marie reported that Color Me Beautiful had solved a simmering family dispute stemming from the fact that she was *cool* and both her sister and sister-in-law were *warm*. As the youngest of the three, she always took their advice at the mall but was later depressed about her purchases, which made her look dull and tired. Her sister and sister-in-law had bullied her into buying tawny tones that looked good on *them*. After Anne Marie realized what her strengths were as a *cool* person with dark hair and dark eyes, she was able to resist their *warm* advice and buy jewel tones.

Alice was distressed because her hair was turning silver prematurely. At only 35, she had no idea what to do about her new head of gray hair. She came for a color analysis asking if she should color it, add red, or get gold highlights. Because she was so young and her brown eyes and silver hair were a striking combination, Color Me Beautiful answered her question quickly and gave her the confidence to stay silver and enjoy it.

Read ahead to solve your own color dilemma!

seeing is believing:
the one-hour makeover

There is no greater testament to the amazing power of color than seeing it with your own eyes. In this chapter you will view a diverse group of women from the same office environment. You will see that every woman, regardless of age, ethnicity, or coloring, can be dramatically transformed through the power of color.

We went into the the office where this group of women worked and set up our photo shoot. The entire photo shoot was done within a single afternoon session. First the volunteers were dressed in their wrong clothing and makeup colors and photographed. Next the ladies were dressed in their right clothing and makeup colors and under the same lighting photographed a second time. They dressed under hurried conditions just as you would in the morning. And as you can see for yourself the results are—in a word—stunning.

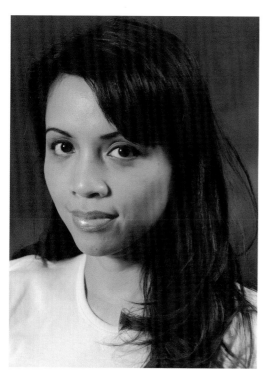

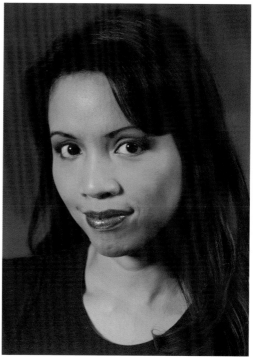

Ira has dark brown eyes and black hair. Anyone with this type of bold coloring looks sallow while increasing the appearance of dark circles under the eyes.

When made up and dressed in shades from her palette, even in a simple tee, Ira is transformed. Her hair looks shinier; her loveliness radiates for all to see.

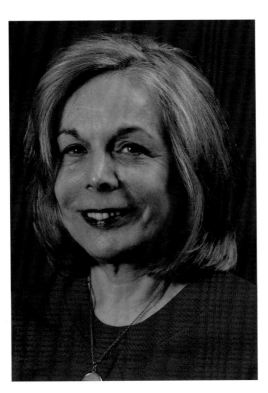

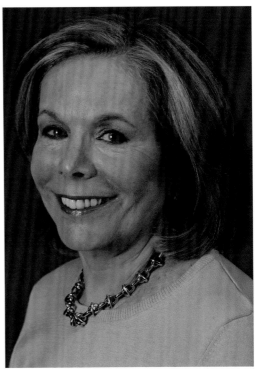

Judy's mother taught her never to leave home without blazing-red lipstick. She also read in a magazine that one of her role models loved the color red, and so she chose it for most of her clothing.

Once Judy is taken out of the red and put into the colors of her season—*cool* pinks and mauves—she is transformed into a picture of sophistication. She loses years from her appearance, and you can see her eyes sparkling.

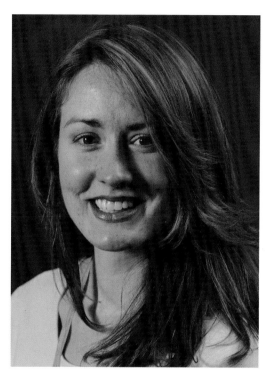

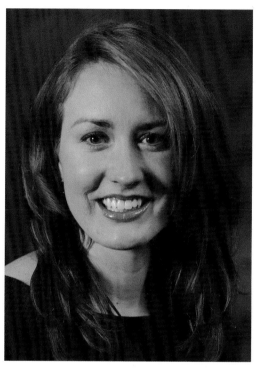

Ashlee had a love of pastel colors, possibly a carryover from her youth when her choices all centered on pink and purple. With a sprinkling of freckles and brown hair with red highlights, *cool* tones pushed Ashlee's all-American good looks into the background.

The moment Ashlee sees herself coordinated in the right clothing colors and makeup colors, her love of pastels is relegated to flowers and baby clothes. Instead of seeing pink or purple reflected in the mirror, she sees herself—the lovely Ashlee, radiant and glowing.

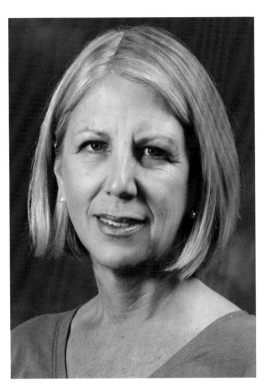

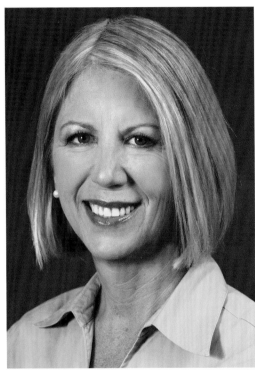

Marianne had been wearing colors that were too intense and jewel-like for her coloring. Although attracted to the pretty color, the blue tones of her blouse were overly *cool* and draining for her coloring.

Surrounded by the light *warm* greens, Marianne looks her best.

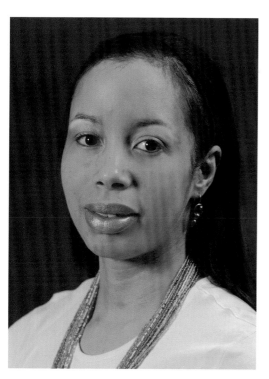

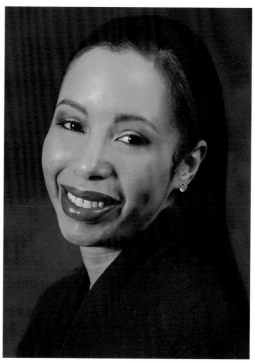

Maiyanna made an interesting observation about the shirt she was wearing—that it looked too plain without the beaded necklace. Often, when an outfit looks as if it "needs something" it's because the outfit is not in your season. Notice how sallow and pale Maiyanna looks in her wrong colors.

In the right colors Maiyanna looks as if someone turned on an inner light. Her skin tone is rich, her smile is lovely, and her eyes are captivating. It's as if suddenly her beauty is revealed.

are you *warm* or *cool?*

Understanding Color Tone to Find Your Season

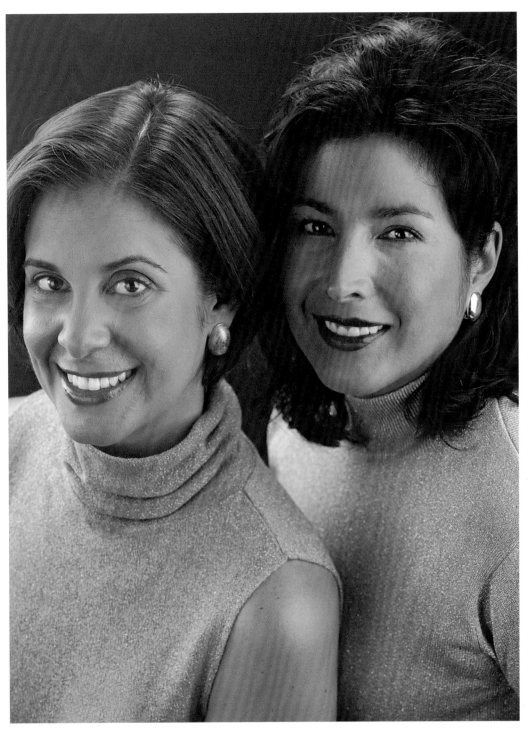

Lisa and Livia

color me beautiful

I n order to determine your season—Winter, Summer, Autumn, or Spring—you first need to identify yourself as either *warm* or *cool*. These new concepts are best visualized. I like to think of them in terms of landscape. After we know your basic *warm/cool* orientation, we can pick your season and fine-tune your colors.

When you envision the *warm* palette, think of a desert panorama. Close your eyes and imagine the brown sand, the burnt orange stones, and the green cactus. Also imagine a pale green aloe plant and a tawny jackrabbit hopping across the salmon-toned creek bed. Now gaze upward, and imagine a turquoise sky with a golden orange sunset.

In contrast, the term *cool* should conjure up a visit to the Arctic Circle. Picture the bluish white ice caps of a glacier and a flock of black and white penguins. Look at the soft blue colors of the sky and sea. Can you see the team of gray Huskies sniffing the cranberry bushes? A silver-gray dusk approaches, then night descends, and the arctic sky turns midnight blue.

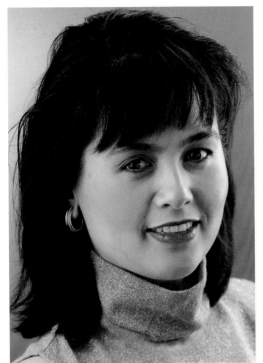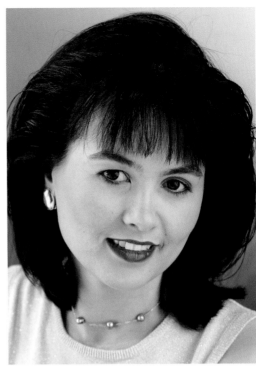

The first step in determining your color concept is to wrap first gold and then silver drapes around your face and shoulders. You would immediately see whether *warm* or *cool* tones looked best on you. When you wear the correct tone, your best features "pop." Your eyes shine, your skin looks smoother, and your teeth appear whiter. The right colors minimize your fine lines and the circles under your eyes. You will soon understand whether your skin tone has gold (*warm*) undertones or blue, purple, or red (*cool*) ones.

color me beautiful

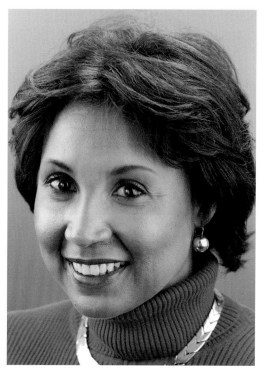 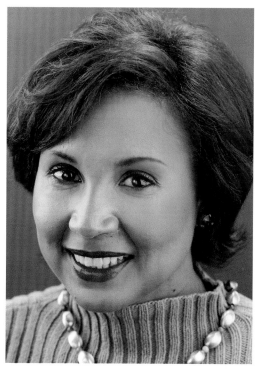

warm or cool?

You are either *warm* or *cool*. The whole key to the Color Me Beautiful analysis is seeing this *warm* or *cool* tone and pulling it together. The goal is to keep it simple and avoid disharmony. Skinny, beautiful, flawless young things on the runway can pull off fuchsia eye shadow and red hair. But most of us aren't runway models and don't have access to their makeup artists. We want people to look at our overall countenance, not our flaws. As we like to say, "What would you remember about this woman if she were running away from the scene of a crime?" Remember this when you analyze your hair, eye, and skin tone.

Stacy's brown hair has many red highlights, and she has dark coppery beige skin tone and dark, *warm* eyes. These *warm* tones do not blend with the *cool* fuchsia turtleneck. In addition, the silver accessories clash with the red tones in Stacy's hair. Look at her makeup—the fuchsia lipstick tends to push Stacy's face into the background. Furthermore, notice how the *cool* blush seems to sit up on her face and does not blend with her *warm* skin tone.

Stacy looks so healthy in these *warm* colors! A moss green turtleneck, amber earrings, and a brushed gold necklace all accentuate her *warm* coloring. Stacy's foundation has a *warm* glow and is finished with a bronzer.

Your Hair

In my experience, hair color is the best clue for determining palette. Consider the hair that you have on your head now, not what you had as a child. *Warm* hair colors have golden and red hues. You are probably *warm* if you can answer yes to any of the following questions. Is your hair red? Copper or auburn? Are you a golden blonde? Do you have brown hair with golden highlights or brown hair with a hint of natural red? Are you gold gray? Or do you have dull brown hair, highlighted with blonde or gold?

warm tones of hair: light to dark

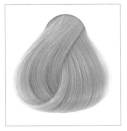
Lightest Golden Blonde

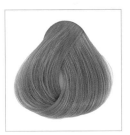
Strawberry Blonde

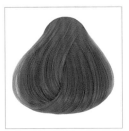
Medium Beige Blonde

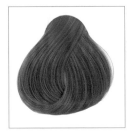
Warm Copper Gold

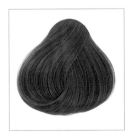
Flame Red

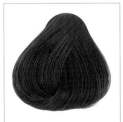
Dark Irish Red

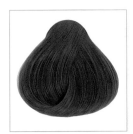
Deep Autumn Chestnut

Your Eyes

Now look closely at your eyes in a mirror near natural lighting. Again, you are looking for *warm* hues. Do you see gold flecks in your eyes? What about brown flecks? Are your eyes amber brown, red-brown, or olive green? Do your green eyes have brown or gold flecks? Do you have blue eyes that lean toward green? Are they aqua or turquoise? If you have blue eyes, do they have brown flecks? Do you see golden brown eyes with green? Are your eyes dark brown? A "yes" to any of the above questions would be evidence that you are *warm*.

Your Skin Tone

It can especially be a bit tricky to discern whether one's skin tone is *warm* or *cool*. For our purposes, the skin tone you inherited is your skin tone. It does not change with a summer suntan or your 60th birthday.

To evaluate the coloring of your skin, look closely at not only your face but also the inside of your wrists where your skin is most transparent. Do you see a skin tone best described as peachy or ivory? Is it golden beige to golden bronze? Do you have caramel, latte, maple, or dark coppery beige tones? Also look for signs of ruddiness, where capillaries are close to the skin surface. This condition appears more frequently in *warm* skin tones. Freckles are also a *warm* clue.

Be forewarned: sallow skin tone is not *warm*. Any season can be sallow. Sallow skin is an unhealthy, sickly-looking yellow. Do not mistake sallow for golden, which is a beautiful, healthy tone. When you meet someone who is *warm*, you will get an overall impression of golden tones. Her hair will have either a golden or red tone to it. A *warm* skin tone has a fair to golden bronze look.

Checklist to Determine a Person with
Warm *Characteristics*

HAIR
- Obviously red
- Blonde with lots of gold highlights
- Golden gray
- Mousy brown with blonde or gold highlights
- Medium brown with red or gold highlights
- Coppery red brown
- Chestnut brown
- Golden brown
- Dark brown with red or gold highlights
- Darkest brown with only a hint of red

EYES
- Look for a warmth, perhaps manifested as golden flecks.
- Golden brown
- Red brown
- Amber
- Olive green
- Blue green
- Pale or clear green

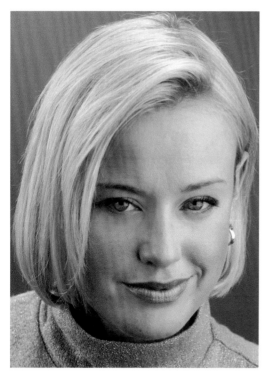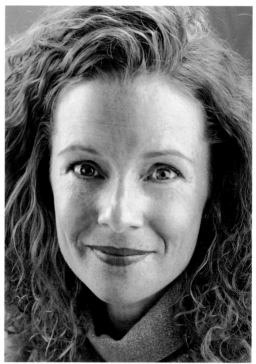

- Green with brown or gold flecks
- Aqua
- Turquoise
- Blue with brown flecks
- *Warm* hazel (golden brown/green gold)
- Dark brown

SKIN TONE

- Ivory skin: Very fair, creamy skin with a yellow/neutral undertone. These tones are common in people with Danish, Swedish, Norwegian, Finnish, and Icelandic heritage.
- Peach skin: Moderately fair, *warm* cream with an orange undertone. Many Northern Europeans fall into this category.

Kristen is a *warm* person. She is able to accentuate her gorgeous natural golden blonde hair, blue eyes, and fair skin by wearing a gold turtleneck and *warm* orange lipstick with bronze gloss.

Look how Susie's eyes sparkle! The gold top and gold earrings emphasize their *warm* golden tones. Her red hair and peachy skin tone with *warm* brown freckles look gorgeous in these colors.

- Golden beige skin: Medium skin with *warm* golden undertones. Often Asian, Mediterranean, and Latino people fall into this category.
- Caramel skin: Golden brown. Many Africans, dark-skinned Asians, Caucasians, Latinas, and Native Americans with golden undertones share this skin tone.
- Golden bronze skin: Dark olive complexion with gold undertones. Golden bronze can be found in Asians, Native Americans, light-skinned Africans, or those of Mediterranean heritage.
- Dark coppery beige skin: *Warm* medium brown skin tone. The dark coppery beige skin tone is found in people with a mixed European and African heritage.
- Latte skin: Dark Caucasian or Latina brown skin.
- Maple skin: *Warm* brown-toned Africans.

are you *cool*?

Your Hair

If you are *cool*, your hair has no red or gold high-lights. *Cools* range from platinum blonde to jet-black. Other *cool* hair colors include off-black, blue-black, brown, ash brown, and ash blonde. (Please note: ash has *no* gold in it.) In addition, your hair may be pearl gray, silver, or salt-and-pepper.

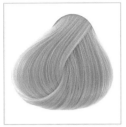
Lightest Ash Violet Blonde

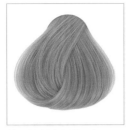
Very Light Ash Blonde

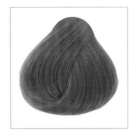
Ash

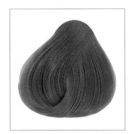
Natural Medium Ash Blonde

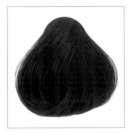
Medium Brown

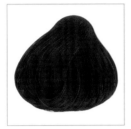
Intense Darkest Brown

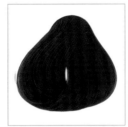
Black with Burgundy

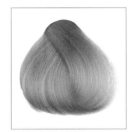
Silver

Two other *cool* hair tones are off-black and jet-black.

Your Eyes

Now look at your eyes. Any gray tones you might see place you in the *cool* palette. Very dark eyes are also *cool*; they include deep black, black brown, or charcoal eyes. If you are *cool* and have blue eyes, they will have white, gray, or only blue tones. If you have any golden tones, you are not *cool*. It's interesting to note that eyes lose the intensity of their color as we age. I have informed many clients that their eyes, which were blue a decade ago, are not now. The concentration of color in their iris has weakened and taken on a gray tone.

Your Skin Tone

Cool skin tones can be confusing because of suntans, which appear golden, and olive skin, which also appears golden but actually has rose or blue or green undertones. Also, any season can have sallow skin tone, which has a yellow tone, or a ruddy complexion. These conditions do not determine one's season.

With these caveats in mind, what is your skin tone? Look at your wrist where your skin is the most transparent. Are your veins blue? Blue veins indicate *cool* skin, which has a little blue pigment in it. Do you have blue or *cool* red undertones? Are you porcelain white? Are your freckles rosy or charcoal gray? Black, olive, and beige skin tones can all be *cool* if they have blue, red, or pink undertones.

The overall *cool* impression is rosy or silvery tones. The hair of a *cool* person has no golden or red tone to it. Her brown will be ash, but her hair can be any shade from ash blonde to jet-black. *Cool* eyes have no *warm* tones to them. If they are in the brown family, they are deep brown. They may also be a *cool* hazel, brown with green or blue; otherwise they are an icy shade of green, blue, or gray. *Cool* skin will have a pink, blue, or red undertone but can be any shade from pale beige to ebony black.

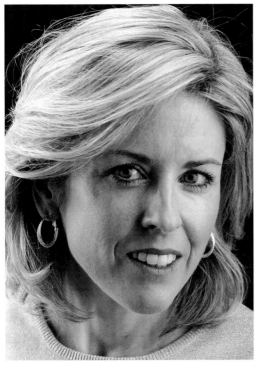 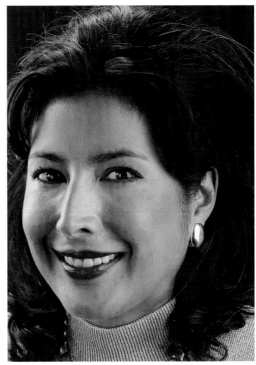

Checklist to Determine a Person with
Cool *Characteristics*

HAIR

- Violet blonde
- Platinum blonde
- Blue gray
- Silver gray
- White blonde
- White
- Salt and pepper
- Ash blonde (often a towhead as a child)
- Ash brown
- Brown with silver and ash
- Medium brown with no *warm* highlights
- Dark brown with or without burgundy highlights

- Off-black
- Jet-black
- Blue black

EYES

- Blue with gray or white flecks
- Soft gray-blue
- Soft gray-green
- Gray
- Dark blue, violet
- *Cool* hazel
- Turquoise
- Green
- Green with white flecks
- Dark brown
- Black brown
- Dark blue

SKIN TONE

- Porcelain: Slight pink undertones. Many people of Irish ancestry have this very delicate skin.
- Beige: Fair with slight yellow or neutral (not golden) undertones. It is a very common Caucasian skin tone.
- Rosy beige: Fair with obvious pink undertones
- Rosy or gray freckles
- Olive: A combination of red, yellow or neutral, and green tones. Many people of Asian, Latin, and Mediterranean descent have olive skin.
- Almond: Light brown skin tone common to Africans, Latinas, and Asians

- Mocha: Light brown with a reddish brown cast. It is a skin tone shared by Africans and Native Americans.
- Cocoa: Medium brown seen in those of African, Latin, or Asian descent
- Mahogany: Medium brown with a reddish-brown cast. It can be found among those of African and Native American descent.
- Ebony: The deepest, darkest brown African complexion. It is almost black.
- Black with blue undertone: An African skin coloring

Okay, you've done the tricky part—but here's an important warning: it is possible to switch from *warm* to *cool* around your fiftieth birthday. When Marian met her husband, he had brown hair with natural red tones and *warm* golden beige, lightly freckled skin. Twenty-six years later, he had changed from a *warm* to a *cool* person. His hair is now over 50% silver, the red is gone, and his skin tone lost its golden beige glow and has became rosy beige. Needless to say, Marian has enjoyed purchasing him a new wardrobe (and hiding those old gold-and-tortoise shell glasses!)

■   ■   ■

You've done the difficult work of figuring out the nuances of your coloring. Now that you know whether you are *warm* or *cool*, let's figure out your season.

the
four
seasons

Adding "Light" and "Deep"
to Your Color Tone

You have completed the first and most difficult step in Color Me Beautiful's analysis. You have identified yourself as either *warm* or *cool*. *Warm* people are either Springs or Autumns, and *cool* people are Summers or Winters.

The only task left to you is to determine whether you are "light" or "deep." If your hair is blonde, light brown, or light red, you are "light." If your hair is brunette, dark red, or black, you are "deep." It's so easy from here:

- If you are *cool* and deep then you are a Winter.
- If you are *cool* and light then you are a Summer.
- If you are *warm* and deep then you are an Autumn.
- If you are *warm* and light then you are a Spring.

winter—color me beautiful's
cool and deep person

Winter's Hair

Winter's gray looks gorgeous and dramatic. Winters are the lucky season and do not have to chemically enhance their hair. If a Winter's hair is all black, it will have no red highlights. These black tones include jet-black, brown black, and Asian blue-black. Medium to dark brown with ash highlights, silver, white, and salt-and-pepper also are included in the Winter palette. You cannot be blonde and be a Winter.

Winter's Skin

Winter has many skin tones. They include porcelain white, beige, rosy beige, olive, *cool* beige, almond, cocoa, mocha, mahogany, and ebony to black with blue or reddish undertones. Many Africans, Asians, Native Americans, Latinas, and Middle Eastern people will fall neatly into this category.

If your skin is olive or light black, look closer. At first glance it may appear golden. However, a *warm* palette will make your eyes appear dull and the skin tone flat, whereas the *cool* Winter shades will brighten the whites of your eyes, and your skin tone will look healthier and more even-toned.

Winter's Eyes

Most Winters have a deep, dark eye color. These eye colors can include black, black brown, and red brown to *cool* hazel with blue or green. A sprinkling of Winters will have dark blue, gray-blue, gray-green, or charcoal eyes. Gray rims around the iris are also a Winter indicator.

Notable Winters

Your coloring resembles Catherine Zeta Jones, Courtney Cox Arquette, Barbara Bush, Connie Chung, Michelle Kwan, Sandra Oh, Condoleezza Rice, Salma Hayek, Penelope Cruz, Ann Curry, and Halle Berry.

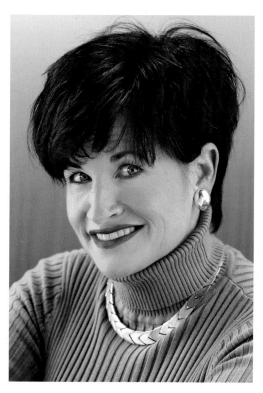

Look how Deedee glows in Chinese blue. Her porcelain skin tone, big blue eyes, and dark hair makes Deedee a unique Winter.

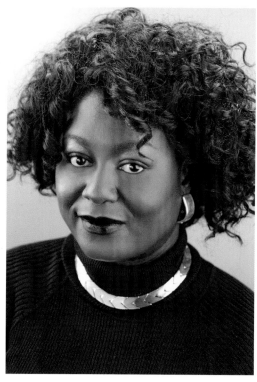

Susie brought her favorite top for this photo shoot. Her skin is ebony without any brown or bronze. Do you see how the whites of Susie's eyes are clear and bright and contrast with her very dark eyes? Her skin appears to have an overall silver tone.

best colors for winter

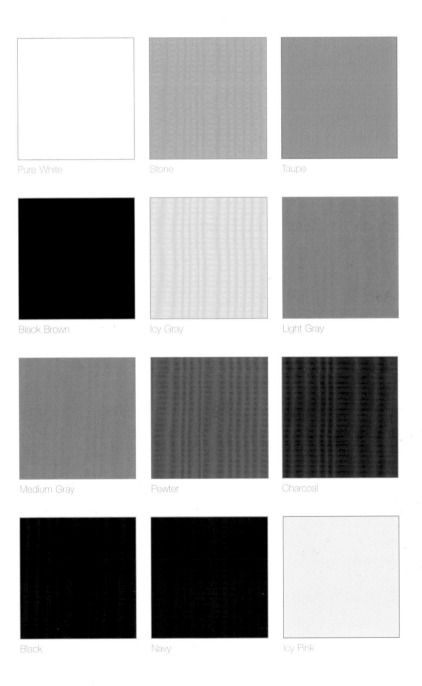

Pure White

Stone

Taupe

Black Brown

Icy Gray

Light Gray

Medium Gray

Pewter

Charcoal

Black

Navy

Icy Pink

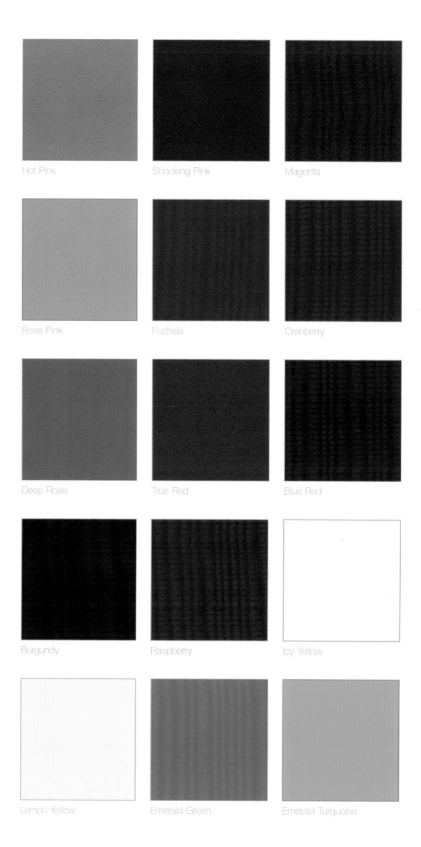

Hot Pink

Shocking Pink

Magenta

Rose Pink

Fuchsia

Cranberry

Deep Rose

True Red

Blue Red

Burgundy

Raspberry

Icy Yellow

Lemon Yellow

Emerald Green

Emerald Turquoise

color me beautiful

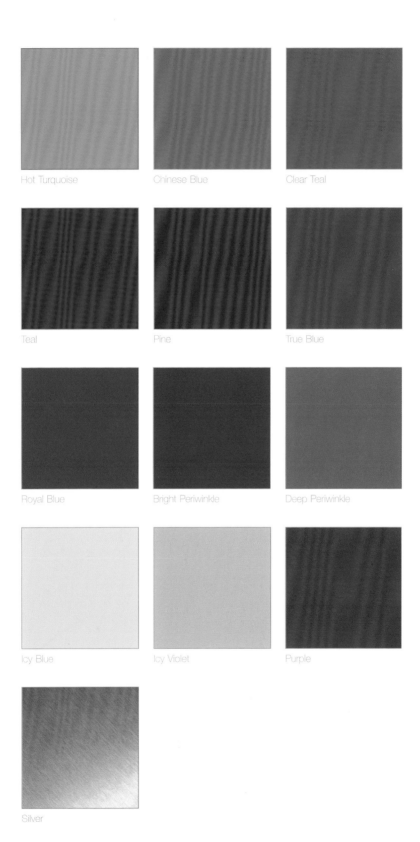

Hot Turquoise

Chinese Blue

Clear Teal

Teal

Pine

True Blue

Royal Blue

Bright Periwinkle

Deep Periwinkle

Icy Blue

Icy Violet

Purple

Silver

Summer's Hair

A person in the Summer palette will either be gray, brown, or blonde. Summer brown may be light, medium, or dark ash brown and will have ash highlights. Summer gray is either pearly *cool* gray or gray blonde. Summer blondes will have no gold to their hair, only ash tones. Many Summers have an overall dusty or muted look. Color Me Beautiful recommends adding contrast to Summer hair with ash highlights.

Summer's Skin

Pink, rose, or blue are the skin undertones of Summers. Skin tones range from the lightest porcelain to pale, neutral, or *cool* beige. Rose beige is also a very common skin tone for Summers. Summers may have pink skin or cheeks. If they have freckles, which is rare, they are charcoal gray or rosy.

Summer's Eyes

There are no brown-eyed Summers. The most common Summer eye colors include blue or green with white flecks, gray blue, aqua, blue green, blue gray, grayish, or *cool* hazel with blue or green. In rare cases, a Summer may have a gray rim around her iris.

Notable Summers

Your coloring resembles Queen Elizabeth, Sarah Jessica Parker, Jennifer Aniston, Diane Keaton, Candice Bergen, Judi Dench, JoAnne Woodward, Jessica Tandy, and Michelle Pfeiffer.

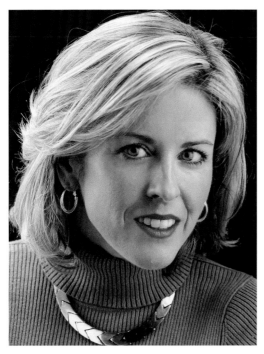

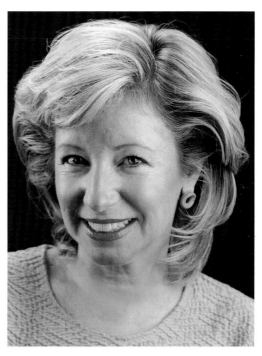

Deidre will certainly receive tons of compliments when she walks into a room in this silvery blue turtleneck, which matches her eyes almost perfectly. Deidre's *cool* makeup, ash highlights, and silver jewelry complete this perfect Summer picture.

Lynn's favorite *cool* pink sweater is a great look for her. The *cool* tones of her hair, green eyes, and rosy beige skin tones make her a Summer.

best colors for summer

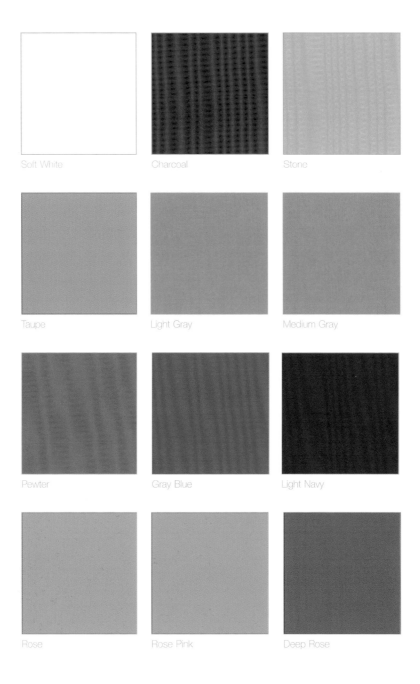

Soft White   Charcoal   Stone

Taupe   Light Gray   Medium Gray

Pewter   Gray Blue   Light Navy

Rose   Rose Pink   Deep Rose

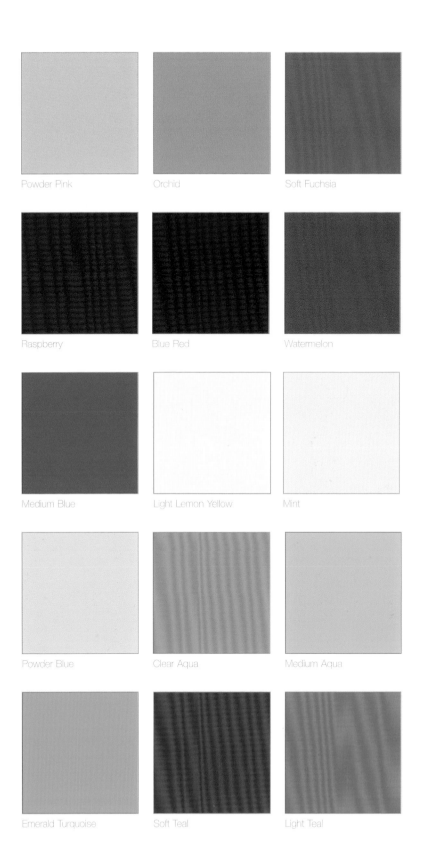

Powder Pink

Orchid

Soft Fuchsia

Raspberry

Blue Red

Watermelon

Medium Blue

Light Lemon Yellow

Mint

Powder Blue

Clear Aqua

Medium Aqua

Emerald Turquoise

Soft Teal

Light Teal

the four seasons

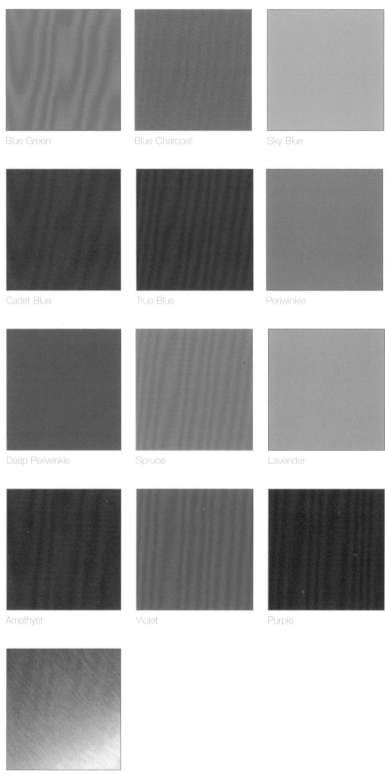

Blue Green

Blue Charcoal

Sky Blue

Cadet Blue

True Blue

Periwinkle

Deep Periwinkle

Spruce

Lavender

Amethyst

Violet

Purple

Silver

color me beautiful

Autumn's Hair

Autumn's hair can range from bright copper red to deep chestnut brown. These tones include golden brown, rich golden red, and dark *warm* brown. Brunette women with a gold or metallic red cast have Autumn coloring. Usually Autumns need to cover their gray because it appears mousy and dull with a yellowish cast. *Warm* blonde or gold highlights are an excellent way to hide Autumn grays.

Autumn's Skin

The skin of a person with Autumn characteristics has golden undertones. These undertones will appear more orange than blue. An Autumn's skin tone can be ivory, peach, golden beige, coppery, bronze, caramel, maple, or latte to golden brown. Ruddy skin is another possibility. Many Native Americans, Latinas, Asians, and people of African, Middle Eastern, and Mediterranean descent are Autumns.

Autumn's Eyes

Autumn eye colors vary to include dark brown, golden brown, green, amber, or an indefinite brownish, greenish color. In Autumns, as in Springs, you will find a golden warmth in the iris. The majority of Autumns have a brown, *warm* hazel with golden brown or green gold tones or have green eyes. Occasionally you will see an Autumn with bright aqua or turquoise blue eyes, and that person generally has red hair.

Notable Autumns

Your coloring resembles Geena Davis, Teri Hatcher, Gloria Estefan, Queen Latifah, Patti LaBelle, Mariah Carey, Jennifer Lopez, Serena Williams, Eva Longoria, Barbara Walters, Julia Roberts, and Beyonce Knowles.

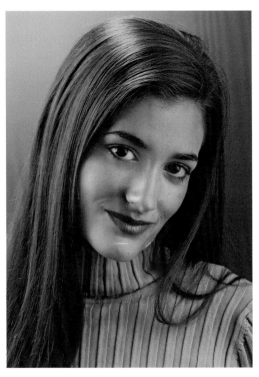

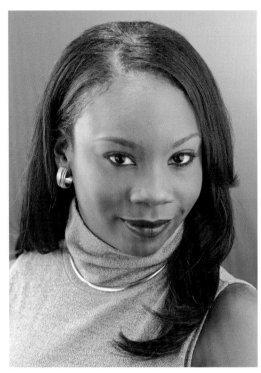

My daughter Julia is all smiles wearing a camel bronze turtleneck. This is an excellent basic Autumn color. It makes her golden bronze skin glow. Julia wears a light bronzer and *warm* eye shadow tones with a gold gloss to boost the *warm* ensemble. Notice how pretty her hair looks lying on her turtleneck.

Khori's brown eyes appear so vivid and clear in her *warm* golden top. Her brown hair with natural red highlights and *warm* caramel skin tone complete her total Autumn look.

best colors for autumn

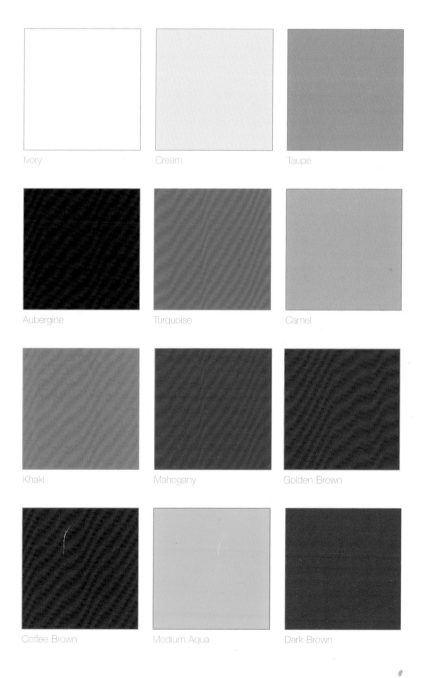

Ivory

Cream

Taupe

Aubergine

Turquoise

Camel

Khaki

Mahogany

Golden Brown

Coffee Brown

Medium Aqua

Dark Brown

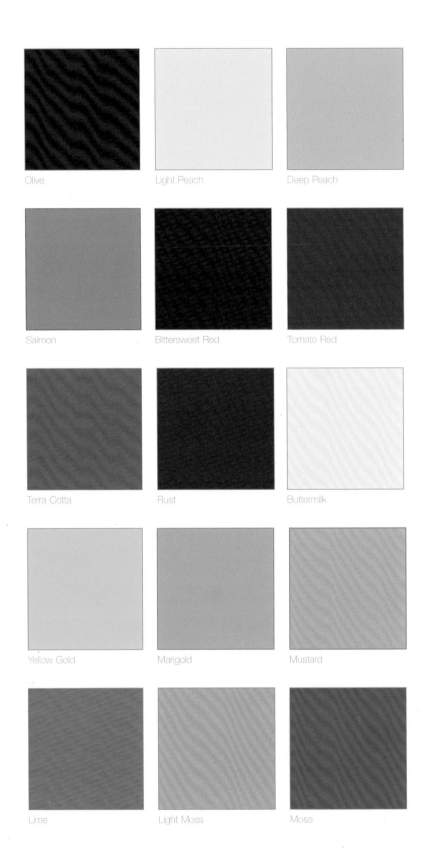

Olive

Light Peach

Deep Peach

Salmon

Bittersweet Red

Tomato Red

Terra Cotta

Rust

Buttermilk

Yellow Gold

Marigold

Mustard

Lime

Light Moss

Moss

color me beautiful

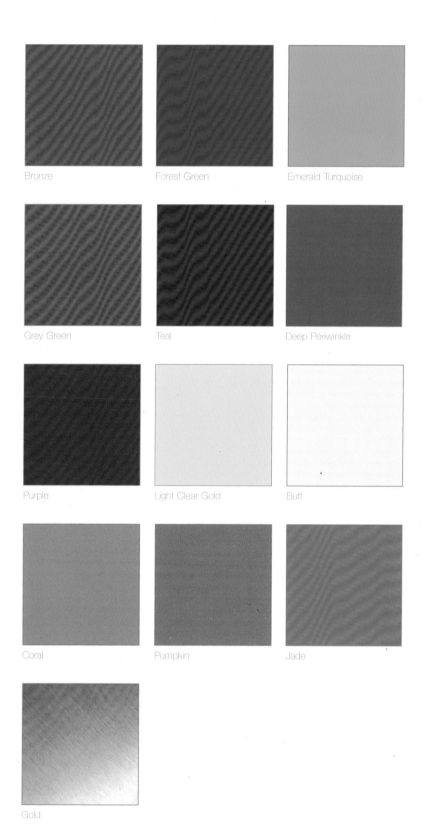

Bronze

Forest Green

Emerald Turquoise

Grey Green

Teal

Deep Periwinkle

Purple

Light Clear Gold

Buff

Coral

Pumpkin

Jade

Gold

Spring's Hair

If your hair is golden blonde, strawberry blonde, caramel, copper, champagne, or beige blonde, then you are a Spring. Mature Springs should cover their gray with the hair color of their youth.

Spring's Skin

The key to Spring skin is a *warm* or golden undertone. Spring skin may be creamy ivory, peach, peach beige, or golden beige; it will always have a delicate look. Springs may have a sprinkle of golden or light blonde freckles. Springs might also have ruddy complexions. Typically Springs and Summers tend to be light-skinned.

Spring's Eyes

The most typical Spring has blue, green, or aqua eyes. Springs may also have *warm* amber, *warm* hazel with golden brown or green gold tones, blue green, topaz, caramel, or turquoise eyes. There may also be golden flecks around the iris. Springs do not have deep brown eyes.

Notable Springs

Your coloring resembles that of Reese Witherspoon, Diane Sawyer, Gwyneth Paltrow, Maria Sharpovia, Nicholette Sheridan, Paris Hilton, Felicity Huffman, or Ellen DeGeneres.

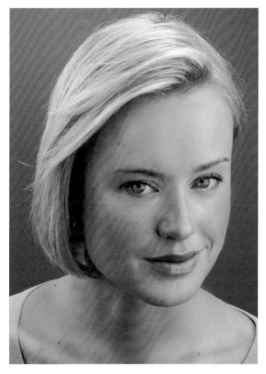 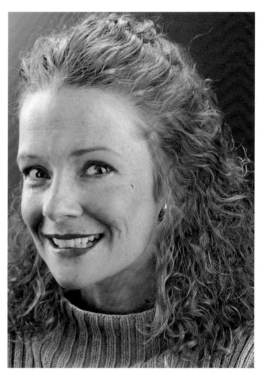

Kristen's golden blond hair, blue eyes, and fair skin make her a Spring. Notice how her skin glows and the whites of her eyes are very clear and bright in this soft peach top.

Susie has unique coloring. Her green eyes place her on the light side of the *warm* palette. Red golden hair, taupe freckles with warm ivory skin and green eyes are three important factors that define Susie as a Spring.

best colors for spring

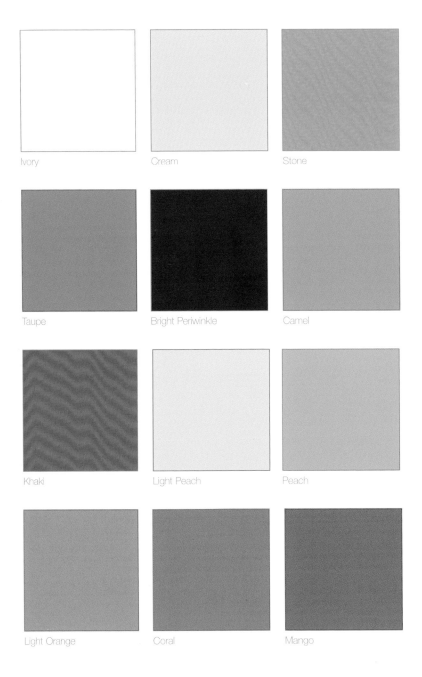

Ivory

Cream

Stone

Taupe

Bright Periwinkle

Camel

Khaki

Light Peach

Peach

Light Orange

Coral

Mango

color me beautiful

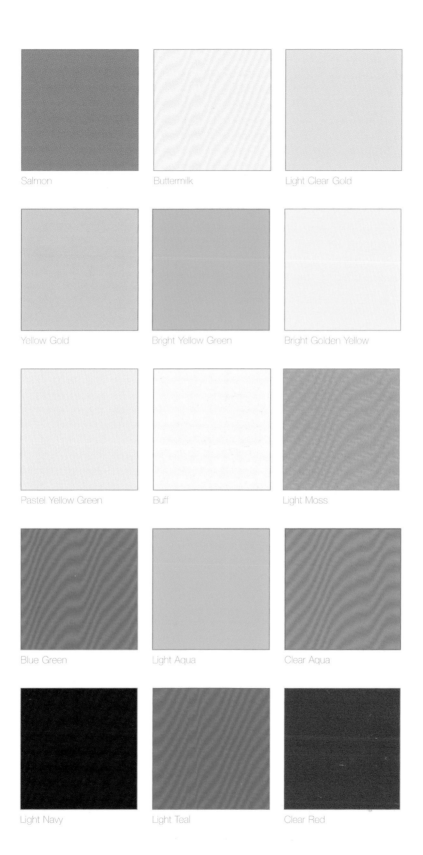

Salmon

Buttermilk

Light Clear Gold

Yellow Gold

Bright Yellow Green

Bright Golden Yellow

Pastel Yellow Green

Buff

Light Moss

Blue Green

Light Aqua

Clear Aqua

Light Navy

Light Teal

Clear Red

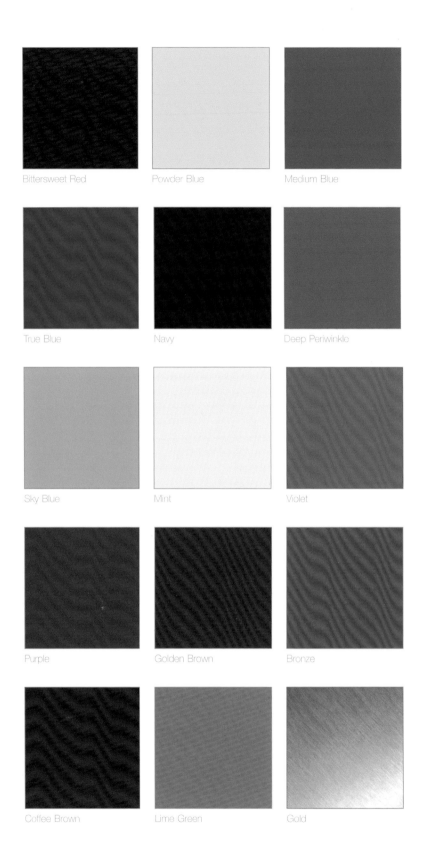

Bittersweet Red

Powder Blue

Medium Blue

True Blue

Navy

Deep Periwinkle

Sky Blue

Mint

Violet

Purple

Golden Brown

Bronze

Coffee Brown

Lime Green

Gold

color me beautiful

Keep these rules close at hand, not only when you're picking out styles for yourself, but also when you're buying for friends who don't share your season.

- Winters are the only ones who can truly wear black and pure white close to their faces and still look and feel terrific. Autumns, Springs, and Summers would feel drained of all color and appear tired in both black and white. If you're not a Winter, you can wear a scarf or accessory in a complementary color and still wear your little black dress.
- A Winter should never wear any shade of orange, brown, or ivory.
- An Autumn should never wear pink or gray.
- A Summer should never wear any shade of orange.
- A Spring should never wear any shade of pink.
- Every season can wear purple.

Now that you have compared seasons and looked at the variation in their colors, you can see how shade and intensity vary between seasons. For instance, Winters and Summers are both *cool*, but one is dark and the other light. Winter choices would be the darkest, brightest, clearest tones, while Summer would be more muted, softer, and less intense.

For example, let's compare the color yellow between the seasons. Winter wears lemon yellow. It is the brightest, boldest *cool* color selection, while the Summer yellow is a softer, lighter lemon yellow. This same concept can be brought to the *warm* palette, Spring and Autumn. Spring yellow is bright golden yellow, whereas Autumn is marigold. Of course, this method can be applied to the other color families as well.

Remember, too, that you can find your palette in nature:

- Winter colors sparkle like a snowflake. They are vivid, clear, primary, or icy colors with blue undertones.
- Summer colors mimic the soft colors of the sky and sea with their *cool* and soft blue undertones.
- Autumn colors are as crisp and colorful as October leaves and have orange and gold undertones.
- Spring colors are like the first daffodil that blooms each year. They have clear delicate colors with golden undertones.

Winter Cool Colors

Lemon Yellow

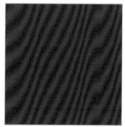
Pine

True Blue

True Red

Summer's Cool Colors

Light Lemon Yellow

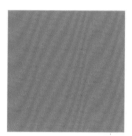
Spruce

Sky Blue

Watermelon

Spring Warm Colors

Bright Golden Yellow

Pastel Yellow Green

Clear Aqua

Bittersweet Red

Autumn's Warm Colors

Marigold

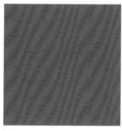
Moss

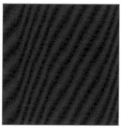
Teal

Tomato Red

the four seasons

COLOR	WINTER	SUMMER	AUTUMN	SPRING
WHITE	Pure white	Soft white	No white Substitute ivory	No white Substitute ivory
BEIGE	Stone Taupe	Stone Taupe	Ivory Crème Taupe Buttermilk Buff	Ivory Crème Taupe Buttermilk Buff Stone
GRAY	Icy gray Light gray Medium gray Pewter Charcoal	Light gray Medium gray Pewter Gray blue Charcoal	No gray	No gray
BROWN	No brown No tan	Rose brown No tan	All brown Camel Khaki Bronze Mahogany Golden brown Coffee brown Dark brown	Coffee brown Camel Khaki Golden brown Bronze
BLACK	Black Black brown	No black Substitute light navy	No black Substitute dark brown	No black Substitute light navy
NAVY	Navy	Light navy	Navy	Light navy

BLUE	Chinese blue	Powder blue	Deep periwinkle	Light teal
	Clear teal	Soft teal	Medium aqua	Powder blue
				Medium blue
	Teal	Light teal	Emerald turquoise	True blue
	Emerald turquoise	Blue charcoal	Teal	Sky blue
	True blue	Sky blue		Deep periwinkle
	Royal blue	Cadet blue		Bright periwinkle
	Bright periwinkle	True blue		
	Deep periwinkle	Periwinkle		
	Icy blue	Deep periwinkle		
		Medium blue		
TURQUOISE	Hot turquoise	Clear aqua	Medium aqua	Light aqua
				Clear aqua
GREEN	Emerald green	Spruce	Olive	Bright yellow green
	Pine	Mint	Lime	Pastel yellow green
		Emerald turquoise	Moss	Light moss
		Blue green	Light moss	Blue green
			Forest green	Mint
			Jade	
			Gray green	
ORANGE	No orange	No orange	Light peach	Light peach
			Deep peach	Peach
			Salmon	Light orange
			Terra cotta	Coral
			Rust	Mango
			Coral	Salmon
			Pumpkin	

COLOR	WINTER	SUMMER	AUTUMN	SPRING
PINK	Icy pink Hot pink Shocking pink Magenta Rose pink Fuchsia Cranberry Deep rose	Rose Rose pink Deep rose Powder pink Orchid Soft fuchsia	No pink	No pink except warm pastel pink
RED	True red Blue red Raspberry	Blue red Raspberry Watermelon	Bittersweet red Tomato red	Clear red
GOLD	No gold	No gold	Gold Light clear gold	Gold Light clear gold
YELLOW	Icy yellow Lemon yellow	Light lemon yellow	Yellow gold Marigold Mustard	Yellow gold Bright golden yellow
PURPLE	Purple Icy violet Burgundy	Purple Lavender Amethyst Violet	Purple Aubergine	Purple Violet
SILVER	Silver	Silver	No silver	No silver

the color me beautiful
color swatch book

The easiest way to ensure that you are dressing right for your season is to use the Color Me Beautiful swatch book. Your season's swatch book contains the forty personal best color choices for your season. It's available from the Color Me Beautiful Web site (www.colormebeautiful.com). Keep it in your purse at all times so that it's handy when shopping!

your skin care

Implementing a Skin Regimen for Every Season

n order for your skin to feel and look great, you need a skin-care regimen that's right for you. Every skin type has its advantages and disadvantages.

If you have dry skin, you are fortunate because you don't suffer breakouts. If your skin is oily or you have a combination of dry and oily skin, you are lucky because you will have fewer wrinkles.

You probably already know your skin's disadvantages, which is why we'll zero in on how to restore it to its natural beauty every day.

simple questions to help define skin types

By asking the following questions, you'll be able to place yourself in your correct skin type.

determining your skin type

Question	Dry	Normal or Combination*	Oily
Do you break out?	Rarely	Occasionally	Frequently
Do you have blackheads?	Few or none	Few in T-zone	Problem
What do your pores look like?	Nearly invisible	Visible in T-zone	Enlarged
How does your skin look one hour after cleansing?	Dry and tight	Slightly tight for first half-hour; some oil in T-zone by end of hour	Oil break-through in half-hour; shiny nose or forehead in one hour
Do you have facial lines?	Showing signs around eyes, lips, forehead	A few around eyes	None or few
Does your foundation melt away during the day?	Hardly	By mid-day or early afternoon	Within two hours of application

*Combination skin can vary, leaning more toward oily or more toward dry, depending upon the individual as well as situation (including time of year, stress, time of month, etc.). Answer the questions based on the way your skin is now; you may have to adjust your skin-care regime as your skin changes.

Now that you have defined your skin type, let's analyze your skin to choose your most effective specialty treatments.

There are three main skin conditions that can be applicable to any skin type. The skin conditions are (1) sensitive, (2) acne prone, and (3) mature or aging.

Skin Condition	Description	Recommendation
Sensitive	Irritates easily and is often red and blotchy. Can have allergic reactions to products and is usually sensitive to the sun, wind, and cold weather.	Fragrance-free and hypoallergenic products. Should avoid exfoliants
Acne prone	Occurs due to the overproduction of oil by the oil glands. Oil that normally lubricates the skin gets trapped in blocked oil ducts and results in pimples, blackheads, and whiteheads on the surface of the skin. Sometimes deeper skin lesions called cysts can occur.	Lightweight, oil-free, and fragrance-free products Antiseptic toners Products with glycolic acid Retinol Vitamin C Medical attention may be necessary based on the type of acne.
Mature or aging	Skin reaches its maturity at 40 and can be any of the four skin types. Mature skin needs preventive maintenance in order to slow down the aging process. Because of hormonal changes, any number of skin changes can occur, ranging from dehydration to loss of elasticity to acne. Genes, environment, facial expressions, smoking, and sleep positions impact how the skin ages. Skin becomes thin and fragile with age and will show fine wrinkles. Prolonged sun exposure causes premature aging, which will result in sagging skin, deep wrinkles, age spots, and leathery skin.	Night cream Eye cream Products with glycolic acid and lactic acid Retinol Vitamin E Vitamin C Exfoliants Sunscreen

understanding skin tone

Skin tone is the color of your skin. It is one of the three key things you should consider in determining your season along with your hair color and eye color.

Put this book down, and look at the people around you. We all have the same basic skin structure, but that's where the similarity ends. An individual skin tone can range from almost pale pink to black. Melanin is the pigment in our individual skin tone that establishes our skin color. There are two types of melanin: pheomelanin (red to yellow) and eumelanin (dark brown to black). Four to six genes determine the amount and type of skin color. Internally, every person has different DNA or genes.

skin of color

The most common skin characteristic that all women of color (African American, Hispanic, Asian, and Native American) share is melanin, the substance that gives the skin color. Melanin offers some protection from the sun's damaging rays. While each of us has melanin present to some degree, the amount differs by individual and by ethnic group. Because of the protective property of melanin, women of color are perceived as having "ageless skin." Actually, as it is for their lighter-skinned counterparts, those with melanin-rich skin have their own unique set of challenges. The following are some of the characteristics a woman of color should be aware of when selecting her skin-care products.

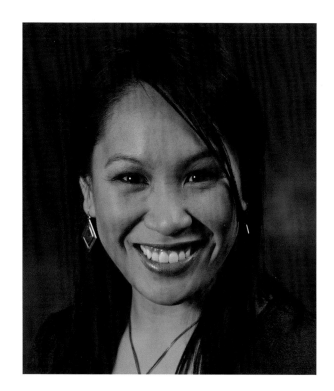

- Women of color have all skin types (dry, oily, combination, etc.).
- Darker skin tends to produce more oil, which can lead to clogged pores, whiteheads, and blackheads. It is important to use products that balance the skin without stripping it of needed moisture.
- Women of color tend to get dryer in later years, but it is also common for older women of color to suffer from oiliness and adult acne.
- Hyper-pigmentation can be the result of an injury, a mild irritation, or acne. It is caused by increased activity of melanin or color-producing cells. Without treatment it can last for a prolonged period.

- Hypo-pigmentation is the loss of pigment, resulting in lighter skin spots. Pimples and scratching can heal to a lighter as well as a darker color. Only a physician can determine whether the conditions are permanent or not.

- A natural phenomenon occurs in everyone as the skin renews itself with the birth of new surface cells and the shedding of old dead cells. These dead cells have no pigmentation and thus are grayish in color. They are more apparent after a bath or quick changes in temperature and humidity. They are more noticeable on deeper skin tone because of their grayish color. A penetrating moisturizer is needed to replenish the skin's natural moisture and to rid the skin of dead surface cells.

- Uneven lip tone, for example where the lower lip differs in color from the top lip, is not uncommon among women of color. In order to correct this uneven coloring, foundation or a special cover stick for lips may be applied under lipstick.

light skin

Light skin lacks protective melacytes and thus tends to be especially susceptible to sun damage and skin cancer. Ultraviolet rays from the sun are responsible for 90% of all visible signs of aging. This is why lighter skin tends to age earlier than skin of color and at a more rapid pace. For purposes of this discussion, light skin ranges from pale ivory to olive. The following are some of the characteristics to be aware of when selecting skin-care products for lighter skin.

- Women with lighter skin have all skin types (dry, oily, combination, etc.). However, the fairer the skin, the dryer it tends to be. This is especially true as it matures.
- The fairer the skin, the more transparent, making it more fragile.
- Fair skin tends to dry out earlier because of sun exposure. Even with sun protection, because of the skin's fragility, prolonged exposure to the sun's UV rays damages the skin.
- Hyper-pigmentation in lighter skin is more likely the result of sun exposure and age rather than injury or acne.
- Fair skin is more prone to rosacea. Rosacea is characterized by redness, pimples, and, in advanced stages, thickened skin. These effects can be masked effectively with a mint-colored foundation adjuster, which neutralizes redness on light skin.
- Fair skin with acne scarring results in red areas on the skin.

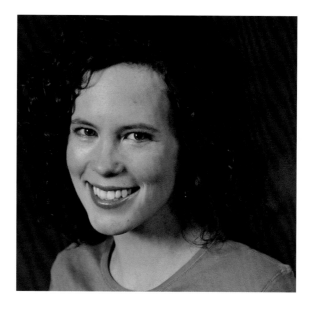

Fair skin like Meagan's can tend toward dryness.

color me beautiful

the ideal skin-care regimen

1. Cleanse daily.
2. Tone daily.
3. Moisturize daily.
4 Utilize specialty treatments daily.
5. Exfoliate weekly.

1. *Cleanse*

Combination Normal-to-Dry Skin

Women with combination normal-to-dry skin should use a gentle cleanser that removes makeup without stripping moisture. Look for the words "rich," "creamy," "milky," or "gentle" on the label. Combination normal-to-dry skin may feel best with a waterless wipe-off or cold cream–style cleansers. Combination normal-to-dry skin should feel soft and supple after cleansing, not tight or dry.

Combination Normal-to-Oily Skin

Women with combination normal-to-oily skin types need a cleanser with antibacterial properties that fight blemishes. This cleanser should also absorb and break down oil while controlling shine. It's easy to forget that harsh soaps and over-cleansing will actually increase oil production while creating unsightly dry patches, so be gentle to your skin. Women with combination normal-to-oily skin types should cleanse their faces when they wake up and before going to bed. Otherwise residual makeup may cause blocked pores. And finally, avoid touching your face if you have combination or oily skin. The germs and dirt that you transfer to your face lead to blemishes.

2. Tone

Combination Normal-to-Dry Skin

Both dry skin and normal skin need the water-binding agents in a well-formulated toner to remove the last traces of makeup and sweep away dead skin cells in your moisturizer. Specialty treatments can penetrate the skin for maximum effectiveness. Toners can also provide antioxidant and anti-irritant protection. Look for toners without alcohol, camphor, or acetone, which can dry out the skin.

Combination Normal-to-Oily Skin

Alcohol toners are too harsh, even for oily skin types. They strip away natural oils, encouraging the skin to produce more oil, actually making the skin more oily. Use a toner with salicylic acid (derived from the bark of a willow tree), because the larger molecule size keeps the product on the surface of the skin, penetrating and exfoliating the pores. It causes the skin to slough off more rapidly, preventing pores from clogging up and allowing room for new cell growth.

3. Moisturize

Apply your SPF moisturizer while your skin is still damp from your toner. By doing this you form a film that locks in moisture. Daily moisturizing primes the skin and makes it easier to apply makeup. Always use up and outward motions to massage moisturizer into your face and neck. This process lifts the hair follicles and enables the moisturizer to reach the top layer of skin.

Combination Normal-to-Dry Skin

The correct moisturizer will immediately improve overall skin appearance, as well as provide long-term benefits. Dry and normal skin types should choose a daytime moisturizer with an effective sunscreen, plant collagen–based nutrients, ceramides, and vitamins. Combination normal-to-dry skin types also need a nourishing and emollient night cream. As you sleep, your skin works overtime to renew itself and repair damage done during the day. A nighttime regimen provides a good opportunity to repair and rejuvenate the skin. SPF is not necessary in every night cream.

Combination Normal-to-Oily Skin

If you have oily skin, choose an SPF oil-free or oil-in-water moisturizer that won't clog pores. These light moisturizers are typically formulated with detoxifying agents and mattifyers (oil-absorbing starch), which give your skin a matte finish throughout the day and keep your makeup fresh longer. However, even with an oil-absorbing product, you may have to use powder to control the shine on your nose and cheeks.

4. Specialty Treatments

Eye cream

Use an eye cream every night and day. The eye area needs special attention because it is the thinnest and most fragile skin on your face. It also has no sebaceous glands, which means that it is more prone to dryness. Apply your eye cream by patting it underneath you eyes, moving from the outer corner toward the inner corner.

Never pull or tug the skin around the eye area. You can find excellent products to reduce puffiness, minimize lines, and lift, tone, and moisturize the eye area.

Lip treatments

Lips also need special attention, whether you live in a warm, dry climate or a cold, damp one. Use a lip exfoliant several times a week to slough away dulling, dry skin. Collagen products will plump up your lips and increase their contour, volume, and moisture. Apply one of these lip plumpers under your lipstick or in the evening as a night treatment. Be sure to use a lip conditioner with an SPF of at least 15 during the day.

Face masks

Combination normal-to-dry skin types should use a moisturizing mask or gel at least twice a week. Masks containing phospholipids are good, for example, but technology changes so often that we can't advocate specific ingredients for dry and normal skin. The best choice for women with combination normal-to-oily skin types would be a refining mask with drawing agents such as mud, sea clay, algae, and honey, which remove oil and impurities from the pores.

Serums

Serums are highly concentrated formulas designed to target particular problems of the skin. They are generally water-based and don't create films, so they can be applied under lipid-based moisturizers. *Glycolic acid* serums increase exfoliation and work well with combination normal-to-oily skin types. *Vitamin C* reduces redness, sensitivity, and irritation. *Vitamin A* works deep within your skin to renew, restore, and repair. *Swiss collagen* helps maintain the skin's elasticity. *Peptides* mimic the effects of Botox and minimize wrinkles.

Skin-tone correctors

Skin-tone correctors are essential for melanin-rich skin tones that are often uneven in nature. You can minimize your skin-tone unevenness and discoloration by applying skin-tone correctors. A recent natural botanical discovery, emblica, is promising to be a highly effective skin-evening and -lightening agent, without any of the negative side effects of bleaching agents. Emblica offers real hope for women suffering from hyper-pigmentation, age spots, and unwanted freckles.

5. Exfoliate

When you exfoliate, you remove the dead surface skin. Exfoliation stimulates circulation and cell renewal, and it provides immediate noticeable brightening and smoothing of the skin. This can be done via a scrub, peel, enzyme, AHA product, or mask. Exfoliating masks are most effective when they are applied to damp skin.

Combination Normal-to-Dry Skin

Surface scrubbing of dry skin can irritate fragile skin, making an enzyme exfoliant a excellent choice for this skin type. A gentle enzyme such as papain, will simply digest the bonds that hold on dead skin, making it easy to just rinse away. Use a gentle hydrator with botanical extracts after exfoliating.

Combination Normal-to-Oily Skin

Exfoliating will make your skin smoother, fresher, and brighter looking. Use a product that will reduce oil-gland secretion, absorb excess oil, and cut down on shine. Since oily skin is less fragile, a scrub or peel will work well. After you exfoliate, deep clean with with algae extracts, clay, honey, or a mud mask.

sunscreens

The most important thing that you can do for your skin is to protect it from the effects of the sun, which can be deadly. The best way to do that is to wear sunscreen daily. Use an SPF of at least 15, and apply it to all exposed skin. By protecting yourself from skin cancer, you will be doing yourself another favor—preventing wrinkles. Some 80% of the skin's visible aging is due to exposure to the sun.

self-tanners

Self-tanners, which come in both sprays and lotions, give a natural-looking glow without streaks if you follow a few important steps. Summers should be the most conservative when using self-tanners, due to their light and *cool* complexions. Gradual tanners that double as daily moisturizing lotions are a good choice for the very fair.

1. Exfoliate your entire body, including your face. This should eliminate a patchy look.
2. Do not apply moisturizer beforehand. Your skin must be dry.
3. Apply a barrier cream between the toes and to excessively dry areas such as elbows, ankles, and

knees. This can be a moisturizer or petroleum-based product.

4. Work upward from the tops of your feet. Move up the legs, torso, and arms until you reach your face. Apply the self-tanner only to a moisturized face and only in the areas that the sun would naturally touch.

5. Self-tanners can be applied in layers to deepen the shade. Remember the bronze rule: less is more.

6. Wash off the palms of your hands immediately. Let the self-tanner set for at least ten minutes before dressing.

Keep this handy step-by-step guide in your purse when shopping for the right cleansers, toners, moisturizers, eye creams, lip treatments, face masks, serums, skin-tone correctors, sunscreens, and self-tanners. Then place it next to your bathroom sink to remind you of the best times and ways to care for your skin.

■   ■   ■

Now you're ready to determine the right shades and styles of makeup—and the best ways to apply them—just for you!

your makeup transformation

Choosing Makeup to Complement Your Season

ow that you have determined your season, this chapter will help you make the correct choices about makeup to complement that season. It provides a visual reference to help you make those choices. Looking at the following pages you will notice that the *warm* palette seasons of Spring and light-skin-tone Autumn are on the left side of the page, and the *cool* palette seasons of Summer and light-skin-tone Winter are on the right side of the page. Spring starts at the top left with lighter, more delicate color shades, and the colors flow down and to the right into the darker, deeper Autumn shades of eye shadow, blush, and lipstick. On the right side of the page, Summer colors begin at the top right with the lighter, brighter shades, and the colors flow down and to the left into the vivid, bold, deeper shades of Winter.

To guide the Autumn and Winters of deeper skin tone, we have included two additional charts to illustrate the strength, boldness, and depth of color that women of deeper skin tone can create for a harmonious, balanced total look. The *warm* shades of eye shadow, blush, and lipstick are on the left side, starting with the lighter shades and continuing into the deeper shades. The *cool* shades of eye shadow, blush, and lipstick are on the right side, starting with the brighter and lighter shades and flowing into the darker shades.

Even if you don't typically wear makeup, don't skip this chapter! You'd be surprised by how young a dash of the right lip gloss can make you look. It is just as important to have the correct makeup colors as it is to have the correct wardrobe colors. Think about it—the wrong makeup colors don't look any better than the wrong clothing colors do. Inside this chapter, you'll also find tips ranging from how to make your eyes look larger to which foundation is best for your skin type.

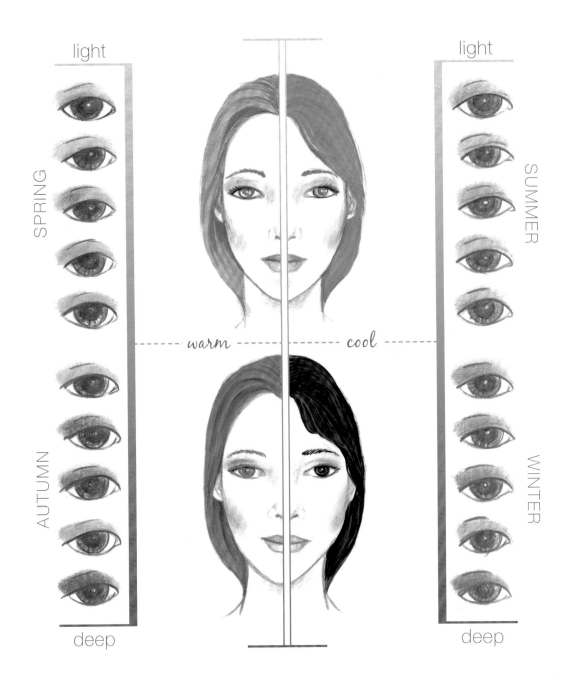

light

light

SPRING

SUMMER

----- warm ----- cool -----

AUTUMN

WINTER

deep

deep

four seasons eye shadow color palette

color me beautiful

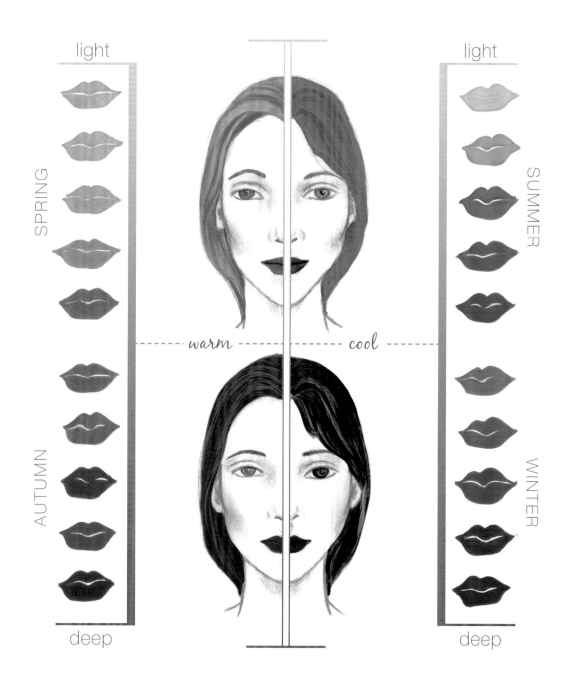

light

SPRING

warm

cool

AUTUMN

deep

light

SUMMER

WINTER

deep

four seasons lipstick color palette

1. Spring's eye pencil colors are medium-to-navy blue, palm green, or light-to-medium brown.

2. Spring's accent eye shadows include light browns, light greens, and copper. Springs can also use a light peach, *warm*-toned highlighter.

3. The Spring blush colors are light and *warm* tones, such as peach, salmon, and light corals.

4. Spring lipsticks are the peach, apricot, mango, and melon shades. Glosses and metallic tones should have a golden quality.

5. Delicate Spring should not wear black mascara. It is too heavy and overpowers her. Brown or navy mascara blend much better.

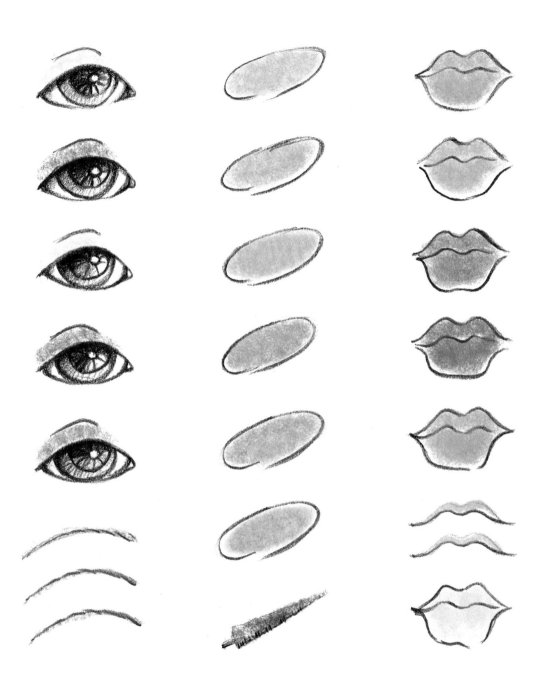

summary sheet for autumns
with light skin tones

1. Autumn's eye pencil ranges from medium brown to brown black espresso.

2. Autumn's accent eye shadows are medium-to-dark brown, medium olive greens, and medium shades of copper. A *warm* candlelight tone is a good highlight eye color.

3. Autumns have a choice of blush colors from *warm* and deep tones of salmon to terra cotta.

4. Light-skinned Autumn lipsticks include deep and *warm* shades of cinnamon, peach, and terra cotta. Autumn's gloss or metallic tone has a gold quality.

5. Autumn mascara is black brown or brown. Save black for the evenings. Black is very severe and will accent any lines and wrinkles around your eyes.

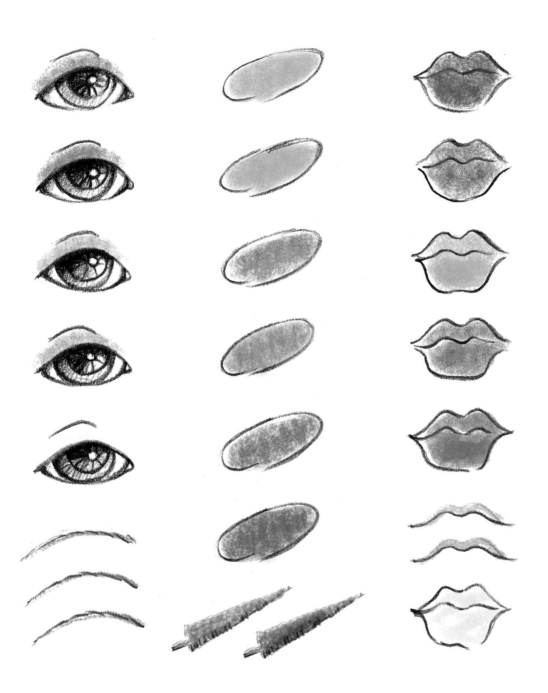

summary sheet for autumns
with deep skin tones

1. Eye pencil shades from dark brown to black suit dark-skinned Autumns.

2. Dark-skinned Autumn eye shadows include chocolate tones, moss and forest greens, and bronze and golden tones.

3. Blushing colors ranging from dark copper, cinnamon, and walnut-to-bark tones suit dark-skinned Autumns.

4. Lipsticks in the medium-to-dark brown family, including sable, mocha, and raisin, flatter Autumns with deep skin tones. The best metallics are bronze and golden honey tones.

5. The proper dark-skinned Autumn mascara is dark brown to soft black.

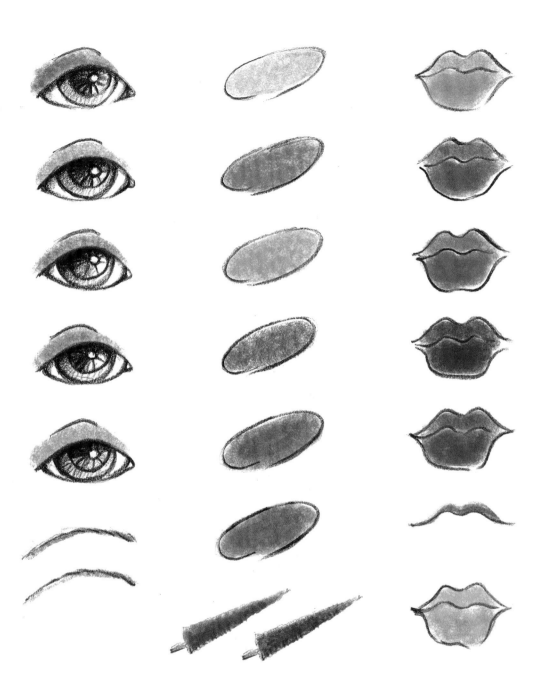

1. Summer's best eye pencils are medium blues, medium greens, and charcoal.

2. The eye shadows that flatter Summers are a mixture of green blue, blue grays, and lavender. The best highlight color is a *cool*, pale pink.

3. Summer blushes include soft pink, rose, and soft plum.

4. Summer's lipsticks are pink, rose, and plum. Summer glosses and metallic tones have a silver shimmer.

5. Navy and charcoal are the proper mascaras for Summers. It is her best choice for day or night. Brown mascara is too *warm*, and black is too severe.

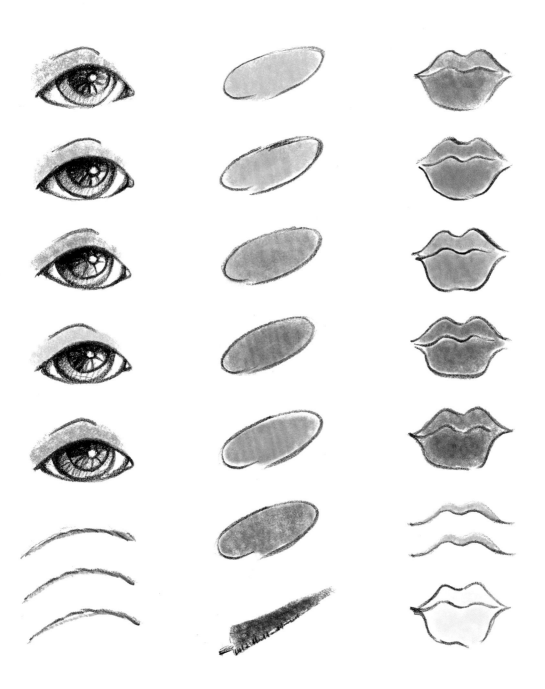

summary sheet for winters
with light skin tones

1. Light-skinned Winter eye pencils include charcoal and navy. Use soft black only during the evening.

2. Eye shadows for light-skinned Winters include medium-to-dark grays, medium-to-dark plums, and medium-to-dark teal. Highlight colors that flatter are *cool*, pale pink, and white with no yellow undertones.

3. Soft red, deep pink, and wine blush colors are the best tones for light-skinned Winters.

4. Hot pink, ruby, bright red, and plums are the best light-skinned Winter lipstick tones. Winters wear silver-toned glosses and metallic tones.

5. Light-skinned Winters should wear navy mascara during the day and black for evening. Black mascara makes the lines and wrinkles around your eyes more noticeable.

color me beautiful

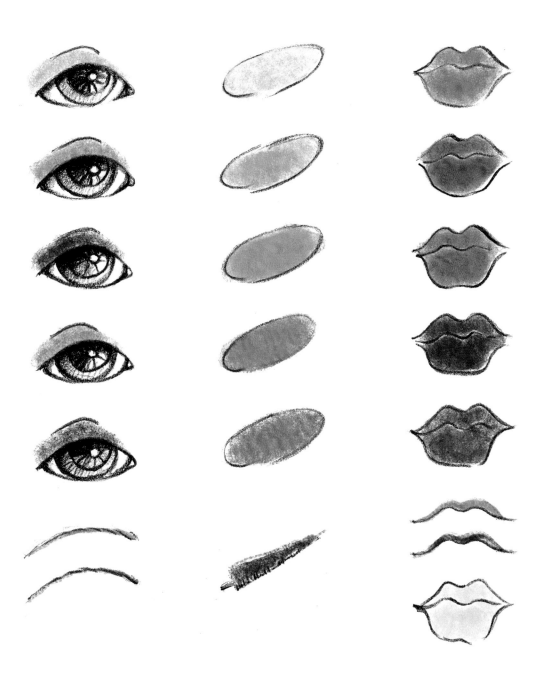

1. The best eye pencils for dark-skinned Winters are black and dark indigo blue.

2. Eye shadows for dark-skinned Winters include deep grays, deep plums, and deep teals. The most flattering highlighter is a shade of medium to deep pink.

3. Blush colors in the deep shades of brandy or cranberry suit dark-skinned Winters.

4. The dark-skinned Winter lipstick shades include black cherry to medium purple tones and deep pinks to rich reds. The best silver metallic-tone lipsticks or eye shadows complement your lipstick tone.

5. Dark-skinned Winters should wear soft black mascara during the daytime and true black mascara for the evening.

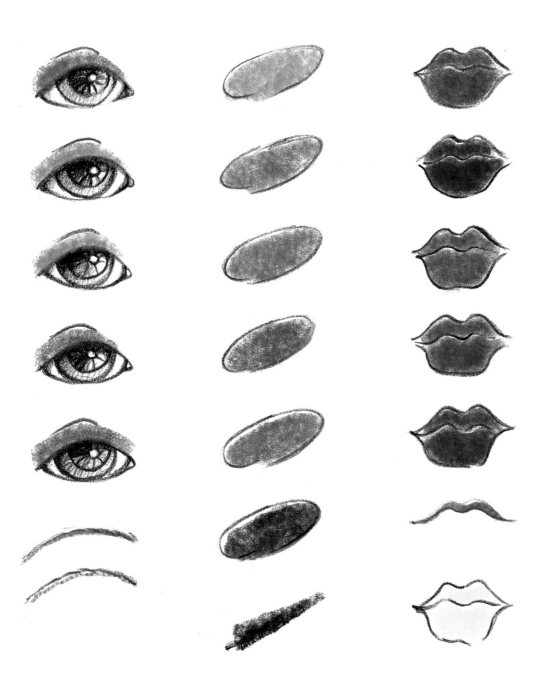

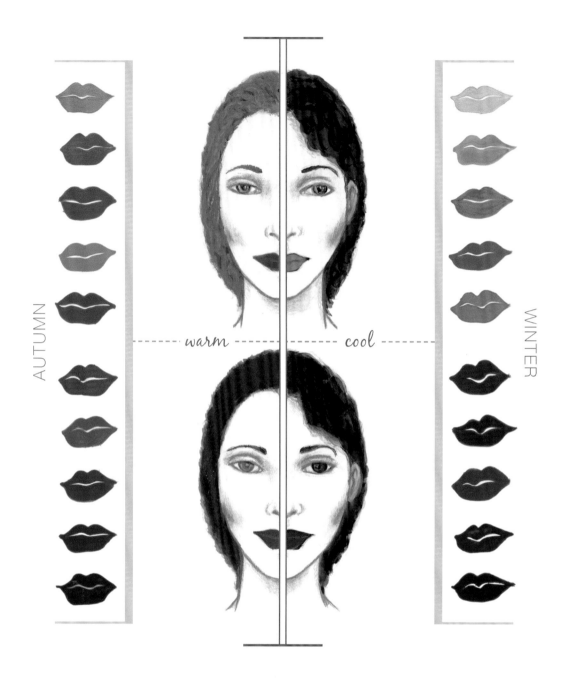

warm ---------- *cool*

deep tone lipstick color palette

makeup application

Refer to the Color Me Beautiful makeup chart for details.

Eye Pencil or Smudgeliner

The Upper Lid

Believe it or not, when eyeliner is applied to the upper lid, it makes your eyes appear smaller. This is especially true with average to deep-set eyes. Prominent eyelids do need eyeliner to make their eyes recede. Unless you have prominent eyelids, only use eyeliner on the outer third of your upper lid and draw as close to the eyelash as possible. This look makes your lashes appear fuller at the base. Beware of liquid liner; it creates a severe look and ages the eye. One remedy is to soften the look with a sponge tip or cotton ball. The end result is a soft, natural-looking eye.

The Lower Lid

To create a soft look on the lower lid, start in the middle of the bottom lid, close to the base of the eye lashes, and extend your line to the outside corner. Then, go back and soften the line with a sponge tip or cotton ball.

Eye Highlighter

Apply eye highlighter before eye shadow. By emphasizing the upper lid with a light powder, the eye is lifted. Apply highlighter from the eyebrow to the eyelid and from the corner of the eye to the outside edge.

Eye Shadow

The primary rule in applying eye shadow is to not apply any dark color to the orbital bone (the orbital bone is the bone on and below your eyebrow). Dark color on the orbital bone makes your eyes look smaller.

Use an eye shadow brush to apply eye shadow along the lash line from the middle of the eye to the outside corner. Don't extend the eye shadow beyond the eye; it makes the eyes look droopy. Now place the eye shadow brush in the crease of the eye, starting in the middle and continuing to the outer edge. Then fill in. Be careful. The purpose of eye shadow is to contour the skin around your eye to either bring out or de-emphasize the delicate contours of your eye. You will find that by creating a base with the mid-tone shadow, the deep tone shadow will go on with a softer and more natural appearance. Re-apply the highlight under the brow bone if necessary.

Mature eyes look younger in a matte or satin shadow that glides on easily. There are two more tips for downplaying wrinkles. The first is to not wear black eye makeup. It is too strong-looking. The second tip is to stay away from iridescent shadows. Both black and iridescent eye makeup emphasize wrinkles.

Mascara

Prior to mascara application, use an eyelash curler. Grip the curler on the lashes for 15 to 20 seconds. When applying the mascara to the upper lashes, start at the root and jiggle the wand up and away. Coat the lashes as close to the root as possible.

Hold the wand vertically when applying mascara to the bottom lashes. Start at the outside corner and lightly sweep the wand across your lashes. Stop at the middle of your eye. Applying mascara across to the inside of the eye makes it appear smaller. Eyes that are puffy, wrinkled, or have dark circles under them are better off without mascara on the bottom lashes.

Average lashes need nonfiller mascara that is highly pigmented. Mascaras with filler ingredients flake and create dark under-eye circles. Mascara lasts for two or three months. Always replace any mascara that is dry or clumps. Never pump a mascara wand; it dries out the mascara formula and increases the bacteria exposure. Finally, avoid curved mascara wands. Mascara is much easier to apply with a straight wand.

Eyebrows

Don't underestimate the power of a well-shaped eyebrow! It can take years off. Think about it: eyebrows frame and balance the face. Shape your eyebrows yourself with a tweezer or tweezing kit. There are also salon professional options: waxing, threading, or electrolysis.

Tweezing Eyebrows

Many women feel it is just better to leave well enough alone when it comes to tweezing. Not so! Bushy eyebrows hide eyes. Follow this process:

1. The best time to tweeze is after a hot shower or bath. Alternatively, apply a hot washcloth to eyebrows for a few minutes before tweezing.

2. Tweeze from the underneath in the direction that the hair grows. Tweezing the top of the brow eliminates the brow's natural arch.

3. It's okay to tweeze the hairs between the brows.

4. Pull hair away from the face. Notice that the right and left eyebrows do not match perfectly. Try to make them appear the same size and shape.

5. Fill in sparse spots with a pencil that matches hair color. Your can also use a lighter shade of eyebrow powder. Aim for a natural look. A drawn-in pencil line looks severe and unnatural.

6. Finish by shaping the eyebrow with a clear eyebrow gel.

Springs and Autumns need golden, reddish, or dark brown eyebrow pencils or powders. Summer and Winter eyebrows look natural with a charcoal or brown pencil or eyebrow powder but cannot use red tones. Keep in mind that pencils tend to go on with more precision and look more defined on the face, whereas powders look softer. Pencils tend to stay on longer, but powders can be set on. And while you have more control with pencil than powder, the latter keeps you from being heavy-handed. This is especially good for Summers and Springs, who tend to do better with powder because their brows are lighter. Use an eyebrow pencil or powder that is a shade lighter than your natural brow color. Eyebrow color should blend well with your hair color. Salon professionals can dye or lighten brows. Eyebrow powders are not the same as eye shadows. Eyebrow powder is drier and duller, and the final result is not creamy or shiny. In addition, eyebrow gel works wonders on unruly brows. A clear eyebrow gel finish gives a polished look.

Concealer

Concealers quickly and effectively disguise blemishes, dark circles, shadows, and scars to make your skin look perfect. They should be applied before you sponge on your foundation. You can also add a second layer of concealer after applying foundation, but be sure to set the second layer with powder. Some concealers are a concentrated form of foundation. These concealers have a lot of pigment and therefore can completely cover problem areas.

Many women mistakenly use too light a shade of concealer. Instead of minimizing eye circles, it produces the "Raccoon Eye Effect," which only makes the dark circles look worse.

The goal of using concealer is to neutralize the flaw before it is covered by foundation. Therefore, use a mint green tone to neutralize red-toned skin found in blotches or rosacea. Yellow will conceal bluish bruises, under-eye circles, sun damage, and pregnancy mask. And lavender neutralizes yellow-colored imperfections, such as sallow complexions and yellow bruises.

Use the ring finger to apply the concealer. The ring finger is the weakest and does not drag or pull on the skin around the delicate eye area. Synthetic brushes work well too. Note that the dried foundation on the foundation lid makes a good substitute concealer.

Make sure to apply the concealer to the recessed inner eye. Put one dot on the area between your eye sockets and nose joint. It creates a wide-awake look.

There are different types of concealer:

1. Cream-to-powder concealer goes on like a cream but dries with a powder finish.
2. Stick concealer is easy to apply; it usually comes in a lipstick-style case. This product is great for pinpointing tiny imperfections. Twist the lipstick container, dot the area to be concealed, and pat with your ring finger.
3. Cream or liquid concealer can be applied with a small brush or your ring finger and set with loose powder.

Foundation

When choosing a foundation, look at its base color. Summers and light-skinned Winters need pink-to-rose tones. *Cool,* dark skin tones need a red base with cognac, espresso, or mink tones. The *warm* skin tone of Springs and light-skinned Autumns blend well with a yellow or golden tone. And *warm* brown skin tones look best in foundations that have a honey, amber, or ginger tone. Also keep in mind these tips:

1. Oil-free and matte foundations are excellent for oily skin. They have no shine when dry.
2. Water-based foundation is for normal-to-dry skin types. It is an excellent product because blush and eye shadows blend with it easily.
3. Oil-based foundations are for extremely dry or wrinkled skin. Their emollient ingredients help the skin look dewy and also minimize wrinkles.

4. Pressed powder base foundation comes in a compact. It performs like pressed powder, except that it provides more coverage. Pressed powder blends easily, lasts all day, and feels light on the skin. It works best on women with normal to combination skin; it is too drying for people with dry or flaky skin.

5. Mineral pressed powders have natural light-reflecting properties that create a soft finish. They can be used either as powder or foundation.

6. Cream-to-powder foundation is a hybrid between pressed powder and creamy liquid foundation. It provides better coverage than a pressed powder base foundation. This product goes on creamy but immediately dries to a powdery finish and thus eliminates the need for powder.

7. Tinted moisturizers are very sheer. While they only offer minimum coverage, they do even out skin tone. Furthermore, tinted moisturizers usually have an SPF of 15. If the color of the tinted moisturizer is too dark, blend it with moisturizer. Tinted moisturizer is a great product to wear when participating in outdoor sports.

Foundation should have a light texture and blend perfectly. It should provide coverage and enhance the complexion, while smoothing out the texture and tone of your skin. To find a perfect match, use your season's makeup guide. Test your foundation in natural light. Apply it along the jaw line. Does the color blend with the color of your neck?

Before applying foundation, cleanse, tone, and moisturize your face and neck. Wait at least five minutes for the moisturizer to be absorbed into the skin. Choose your foundation based on your skin type (dry, normal, combination, or oily).

Apply foundation with a wedge-shaped sponge, your clean fingers, or a makeup brush. For sheer coverage, dampen the sponge. If the foundation comes in a compact, apply it with the included sponge. Apply cream and liquid foundations with your fingers or a wedge-shaped sponge. A big brush is the best way to apply loose powder foundation.

Some of us may need two foundations to combat uneven skin pigment. To apply two foundations, put the shade that matches your jaw line in a circle around your face and near your hairline. Then blend it in toward the center of your face. Next, apply one shade lighter on the planes of your face that the sun would naturally touch. This gives your face some illumination as well as contour. This technique is particularly effective on darker skin tones. The darker your skin tone, the more melanin in your skin, which makes it more likely to be uneven. By applying foundation as described, you'll find that it evens out your skin tone, making your skin appear flawless.

If don't want to use the two-color foundation approach, you can use lighter powder instead. But avoid using blush in a circle around your face. And do not wear foundation one shade darker to give the impression of a suntan. If in doubt between two shades, choose the lighter one. It supports the goal to lighten and lift.

Blush

There are three forms of blush:

1. Cream blush has a dewy finish. It is a good match for mature women with normal to dry skin because it doesn't highlight wrinkles.
2. Powder blush works well on all skin types. It produces great results on oily skin.
3. A gel blush creates a sheer, translucent glow and is long lasting, but it is difficult to blend into dry skin.

To apply blush, start mid-cheek, about as far in as your pupil is, and apply from your cheekbone to your hairline. Blend downward to soften. Don't apply too high, or the blush will encroach on your eye area. However, blush below your cheekbone makes you look drawn and tired. Apply the blush after concealer and foundation. Blush color depends on skin tone, of course. Pick the best one for your season from the makeup chart.

Lip Pencil

Lip pencils or lip liners keep lipstick from bleeding beyond the edges of our lips. The wicking process of drier skin draws emollients from lips and pulls color into lines around our lips. Because lip liner has no emollients in it, it's an effective barrier.

You may want to use a concealer or your foundation to cover your lips and form a base before using a lip pencil. Line your natural top and bottom lip ridge. Then color in your entire lip with the pencil. This gives your mouth definition, and your lipstick will stay on longer. Young women who don't want to wear lipstick yet could use a lip pencil in their season topped off with clear gloss. Lip liners are necessary for mature women. As we age our lip line becomes thinner and less defined.

Dark-toned lip pencils make lips look larger, and lighter tones make them appear smaller. Lip pencils should be the same color or slightly darker than your lipstick. Refer to the makeup chart to select the best lip liner colors for your season.

Lipstick

Every woman should use lipstick, because, as we age, our lips begin to lose their color. Don't leave home without your lipstick! Here are some lipstick facts to remember. Matte lipstick is dry but lasts a long time. Cream lipstick is more emollient than matte. Highlighting or sheer lipsticks tend to bleed. While gloss lipstick is very moist, it does not stay on as long as other formulas. Women who have problems with their lipstick feathering should stay away from lip glosses and always use a lip pencil. Metallic-toned lipstick looks best on women younger than 25. It highlights lip wrinkles.

Make sure that your lipstick color harmonizes with your clothes. Mature women should avoid dark lipstick shades, which are aging, as well as lipstick shades that are too soft and make you look washed out. The best seasonal makeup choices can be found on the Color Me Beautiful makeup chart.

Lip exfoliation removes dead skin cells and improves circulation, so don't forget your lips when you scrub your face. If you like, use a lip-plumping product before applying lipstick. These new products give lips a base coat of foundation and make your lips appear fuller and softer. Before applying lipstick, remedy uneven lip tone with a cover cream.

Use a sable lip brush to apply your lipstick. After getting color on the brush, paint the upper lip. Begin at the center of the upper lip and follow the left lip line, then repeat from the center to the right. Do the same on the bottom lip. Lipstick has more staying power when it is blotted after the first coat is applied. Reapply and blot a second time for a deeper color.

Apply lip balm before lipstick for dry lips. Let the lip balm absorb thoroughly before applying lipstick. In addition, it is important to protect and condition lips from the sun, wind, and cold. So use a lip balm with an SPF factor.

■   ■   ■

These makeup tips and tricks, paired with your new seasonal makeup color choices, will take your look up to a whole new level. Use our suggestions to look and feel your most confident.

your best
hair color for
your season

Making Choices with Your
Seasonal Palette in Mind

I f you highlight your hair or cover your gray, keep your entire seasonal palette in mind when you make hair-color decisions. By following these seasonal recommendations, your new hair color will blend rather than clash with your clothes and makeup. Always remember these basic tenets: Winters and Summers should never add *warm* highlights to their hair, and Autumns and Springs should never add *cool* ones. The palettes that follow represent the actual range of hair colors for any season rather than just the highlights.

winter's deep and *cool* hair

The contrast between Winter's dark hair and silver hair is striking. If a Winter woman does not want to show off her new silver look, she must use *cool* ash brown tones to cover her gray. Do not purchase anything with the word "warm" on the label.

Take Natalie, for example. Natalie was a perfect Winter in all aspects except her new hair color. She had used a *warm* auburn hair dye, which completely undermined Natalie's *cool* look. Once her color analysis was complete, she realized that she needed a hair color that blended with her seasonal coloring. She now looks stunning in her dark ash brown hair.

Mia, a beautiful young Winter with black hair, wanted to highlight her hair. After reviewing her season's colors, she eliminated blonde and red from her choices, because they are *warm* colors. She also found out that if she used peroxide on her black hair, it would turn orange red. The highlights would ruin her *cool* look. One option Mia had not considered was the addition of burgundy highlights. Burgundy is a *cool* color. She added it to her hair and stayed in her *cool* palette.

WINTER'S HAIR

- Medium brown
- Dark ash brown
- Dark brown
- Darkest brown
- Intense darkest brown
- Off-black
- Jet-black
- Blue black
- Silver
- Salt-and-pepper

Examples of Winter's Hair

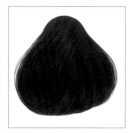

Medium Brown (no gold or red tones)

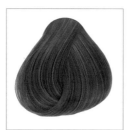

Dark Ash Brown

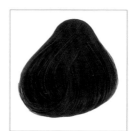

Dark Brown

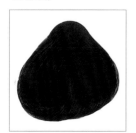

Darkest Brown

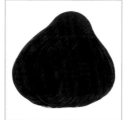

Intense Darkest Brown

summer's ash hair

The natural ash hair that many Summer women have looks elegant. Its muted look meshes nicely with this season's soft look. Summer women need to beware of adding *warm* highlights to their hair. Ash is preferable, whether you are covering gray or just brightening your face. Ash highlights have no gold tones.

Connie, a Summer who was about to turn 50, was upset about her silver hair. She had tried to cover the silver with red highlights, but the new color caused her appearance to lose its equilibrium. Connie's hair was *warm* red, her skin was *cool* pink, and her eyes were a *cool* gray blue. After a color analysis, she removed the red and added ash highlights to blend with her silver. She found balance within her season.

SUMMER'S HAIR
- Lightest ash violet blonde
- Lightest ash blonde
- Very light ash blonde
- Light ash blonde
- Soft pearl ash
- Ash
- Natural medium ash blonde
- Medium ash blonde

Examples of Summer's Hair

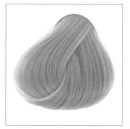

Lightest Ash Violet Blonde
(no gold at all)

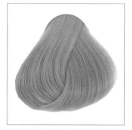

Lightest Ash Blonde

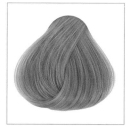

Very Light Ash Blonde

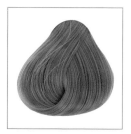

Light Ash Blonde

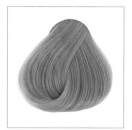

Soft Pearl Ash

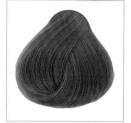

Ash

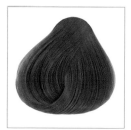

Medium Ash Blonde

autumn's deep and rich hair

Gray hair often comes in dull or yellow on Autumns. Red or gold highlights will lighten the gray in a natural-looking way. Darker Autumns can achieve a beautiful look and cover their gray by coloring their hair to its original deep color.

Maxine, an Autumn, caught her reflection in a mirror at the grocery store and thought, "That blonde lady is wearing the same outfit as I am. . . ." Then she realized she was looking at herself! It never occurred to her before that her highlights had multiplied into a full head of golden blonde hair. But Maxine had not transformed into a Spring. Because she has dark eyes, she remains an Autumn. She will, however, need to fine-tune her wardrobe and makeup to reflect a softer side of Autumn. Softer Autumns should not wear colors that are deep or dark.

AUTUMN'S HAIR

- *Warm* copper gold
- Golden blonde brown
- Flame red
- Deep copper gold
- Rich autumn red
- Deep autumn chestnut
- Dark Irish red
- Dark brown

Examples of Autumn's Hair

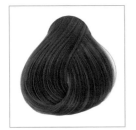
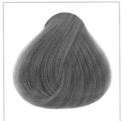
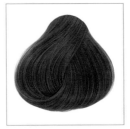
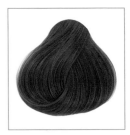

Warm Copper Gold	Golden Blonde Brown	Flame Red	Deep Copper Gold

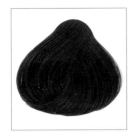
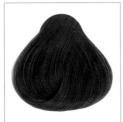
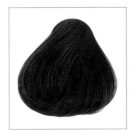
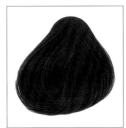

Rich Autumn Red	Deep Autumn Chestnut	Dark Irish Red	Dark Brown

color me beautiful

spring's golden hair

Gold and copper highlights look perfect with the Spring complexion. Never add ash to Spring hair; ash is *cool*, and Spring coloring is *warm*.

Claire was a Capitol Hill attorney. She chose drab brown hair to cover her gray hair because of the conservative nature of her job. But with her bright green eyes and her *warm* skin tone, her hair was just screaming for golden highlights. At first, Claire balked at the idea of showing up to work as a blonde bombshell. But she registered the difference as she incrementally added *warm* blonde highlights. At each hair appointment, she would add a few more, until eventually she became a dazzling golden blonde, with an amazing amount of contrast. Best of all, she managed the transformation with such subtlety that her co-workers merely told her that she looked years younger. No one ever asked Claire, "What did you do to your hair?"

SPRING'S HAIR
- Lightest golden blonde
- Light beige blonde
- Strawberry blonde
- Soft velvet blonde
- Light golden blonde
- Soft caramel
- Medium beige blonde
- Medium golden blonde

Examples of Spring's Hair

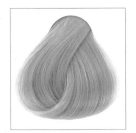

Lightest Golden Blonde

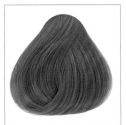

Light Beige Blonde

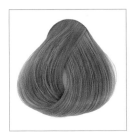

Strawberry Blonde

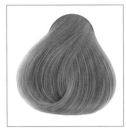

Soft Velvet Blonde

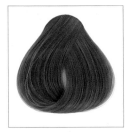

Light Golden Blonde

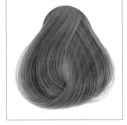

Soft Caramel

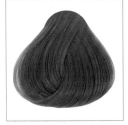

Medium Beige Blonde

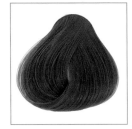

Medium Golden Blonde

understanding your wardrobe palette

Choosing Clothes to Wow the Crowd

How often do you find yourself standing in front of your well-packed closet thinking, "I don't have anything to wear!"? You are not alone—80% of women wear only 20% of the clothes in their closets. Yet we continue to spend our hard-earned money on clothes we do not wear because we don't have the knowledge to make the right purchases or pull out of our closet what's best for our look.

Wouldn't you like to have a closet full of clothes you actually wear? Since the color you wear reflects onto your face, it can enhance your look or detract from it. In order to build an efficient wardrobe, we will use your Color Me Beautiful color swatch book and focus on your seasonal colors. When you shop with your swatch book, you will find that you *can* walk away from a sale item that is not in your palette. The beauty of building your wardrobe around your season's colors is that you have eliminated the negative items. And so doing, you have given yourself a present of a little more money and a little more time.

Juanita, a Winter, had held onto a rust-colored ski jacket that her husband had given her for Christmas years ago when they were newlyweds. She had never worn rust before, but she accepted the gift graciously. She barely wore the jacket, however, and realized when her colors were analyzed that her husband had bought her the rust jacket because *he* was an Autumn. She found out the hard way that you should give your husband your color swatch card before gift-giving time!

winter . . . color me— deep and *cool*

The most vibrant *cool* colors flatter Winter women, who also wear contrasting colors well. They are the only season that can wear pure white, which is often seen against a contrasting shade. Winters are dazzling in intense royal blues, hot pinks to deep fuchsia, and blue and true reds. Winter women can be bold and dramatic whether they are playing tennis or attending a cocktail party.

summer . . . color me— light and *cool*

For Summer women the keywords are soft and sexy. Summers are luminous in complex tones of blue charcoal, lavender, and soft fuchsia, which are *cool* yet very soft. If you are a Summer, choose navy over black in everything from suits to mascara. Avoid pure white, orange, and gold, very dark and very bright colors. These colors can overpower the delicate Summer woman's hair and complexion. Muted, dusty, and hazy colors give Summer women a special glow.

autumn . . . color me—
deep and *warm*

At the risk of stating the obvious, the Autumn woman looks radiant in Autumn tones, with coloring rich enough to rival nature when she is at the pinnacle of her glory. The Autumn woman should steer clear of pure white and favor ivory, cream, or camel and should avoid *cool* colors as well. A good rule of thumb is if you would never see it in the landscape of a crisp autumn afternoon, it probably isn't for you. Olive, tan, and bronze form an excellent foundation for an Autumn wardrobe.

spring . . . color me—
warm and light

Spring women have warmth and delicacy of coloring. They have an entire range of clear and bright tones to show off their beauty. Spring women look great in vibrant shades including salmon, light orange, and bright yellow green. Bronze, bright periwinkle, and peach are other great choices that show off Spring's hair and eye color.

Springs should avoid wearing pure black or white near or around the face, because these colors contribute to a wan and unhealthy appearance. Opt instead for a scarf, blouse, or jewelry that reflects the beautiful selection of bright and clear blues, teals, mints, violets, golden yellows, salmons, and corals with which you can brighten up your basic black suit.

a note on neutrals

Color Me Beautiful separates your swatch book into neutral and basic colors. The basic colors are the more fun colors in your swatch book. But neutrals form the foundation of your wardrobe because they go with everything. Use the following chart as a planning guide:

	WINTER	SUMMER	AUTUMN	SPRING
NEUTRALS	White	Soft white	Ivory, Creme	Ivory, cream
	Black	Grayed navy	Beige	Clear beige
	Navy	Blue gray	Camel	Camel, tan
	Gray		Dark brown	Golden
	Taupe		Gold	brown
			Bronze	Clear gold
			Olive	Light clear
				navy
BASIC COLORS	Burgundy	Burgundy	Forest green	Clear red
	Blue red	Raspberry	Moss green	Orange red
	True red	Gray blue	Orange red	Coral
	True blue	Deep blue green	Bittersweet red	Periwinkle
	True green	Blue red	Rust	Rust
	Emerald green	Watermelon		
	Pine green			

what about plaids and prints?

To determine the season of a particular plaid or print, pay attention to the first color that catches your eye. That dominant color establishes whether the print or plaid is from the *warm* or *cool* palette. A few exercises follow.

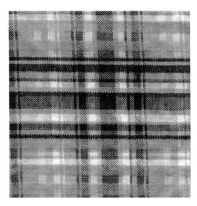

You are shopping and this bright plaid catches your eye. Should you buy it? Do you think that it is a *warm* or *cool* plaid? It is *cool*. The dominant color is a *cool* red with lots of pink.

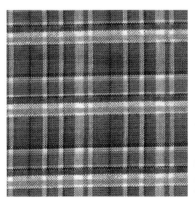

Do you see *warm* orange or the hot *cool* pink? The orange definitely overpowers the pink. You are looking at a *warm* plaid.

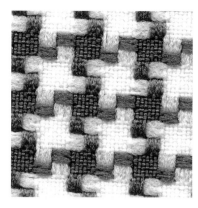

Hot pink houndstooth is a *cool* combination.

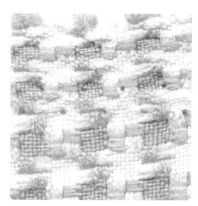

This salmon houndstooth is perfect for a *warm* person.

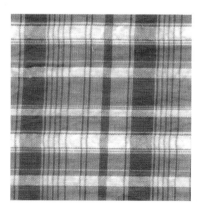

The overall impression of this plaid is orange. There are *cool* purple and yellow stripes, but the dominant color is orange, and it is *warm*.

understanding your wardrobe palette   117

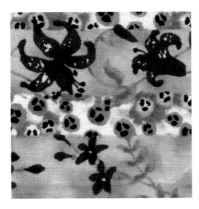

The tan background is *warm*, and the red flowers are a tomato orange red. This print would look stunning on a *warm* person.

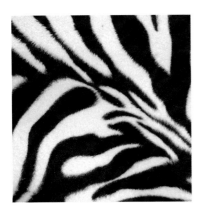

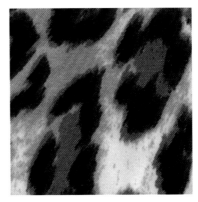

This leopard print's brown and tan tones are *warm*. Alternatively, the black and white zebra print is a *cool* print.

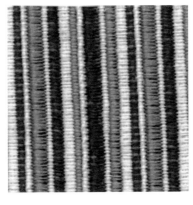

This fun stripe's colors are beautiful *warm* tones, rust and orange.

Now you are on your way to buying new and organizing old clothes that always work and always look good. We have identified exactly which colors form the best foundation for your new working wardrobe. And in the next chapter, you will learn not only about the right accessories for your look but also about how they can help out old outfits as you begin to build your new wardrobe. The last chapter identifies exactly which pieces of clothing must be standard in every woman's closet.

accessories

the finishing touches

If you noticed that last year your season's red was called "Chinese red" and that this year it's "fire engine red," don't be confused. To boost sales, designers rename colors occasionally. Often, only the color's name has changed.

But if one season you find that the "new" reds are slightly bluer, say, than the red you feel most comfortable in, don't worry. There's a solution: accessories.

Earrings, necklaces, pins, scarves, hats, eyewear, and hair accessories allow you greater latitude in your look. And they can be a big help in fine-tuning the color palette of an outfit.

This chapter will show you how to get more out of your closet by accessorizing. It will also help you to make your next purchase in your season.

jewelry

Jewelry is the universal accessory. Earrings and necklaces adorn both your hair and face and can be simple or ornate. Even if you're just dashing out to the grocery store, earrings always take your sophistication up a level. They can change a nice look into a fabulous one. Based upon previous recommendations, you've probably made the leap that your earrings and necklaces need to reflect your *cool* or *warm* attributes. If you are a Summer or a Winter woman, wear silver tones. *Warm* golden tones fight a *cool* woman's skin tone and do not blend. The opposite is true of Springs and Autumns. They need yellow gold tones to blend with their skin.

You may have realized that some or all of your jewelry is the wrong metal. A possible fix is to ask a jeweler to dip your gold jewelry, for example, in white gold. Check with your jeweler about gold dipping as well. You can also find many inexpensive, colorful jewelry options online, through catalogues and the shopping networks and in jewelry stores. Make sure that earrings and necklaces blend with your features and clothing so that you can wear them daily. In the next section, we'll look at the right gems for your best metals as well. This is especially important when making pearl-buying decisions, because these gifts from the sea come in a variety of subtle shades.

a winter woman's jewelry

- *Best metals,* either brushed or shiny, are platinum, white gold, silver, or pewter.
- *Precious and semi-precious stones* include black diamonds, pink tourmaline, rose quartz, sapphire, ruby, and lapis.
- *Accent stones* are garnet, onyx, and rubelite.
- *Clear stones* are diamonds, white topaz, moissanite, and cubic zirconia, which are best set in white gold or platinum.
- *Pearls,* whether real or faux, should have a white, platinum, pink, or silver overtone.

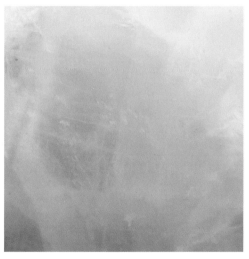

Rose Quartz

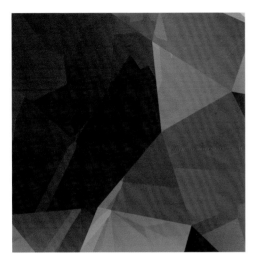

Ruby

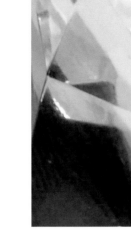

Diamond

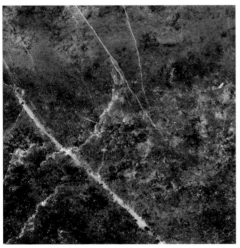

Lapis

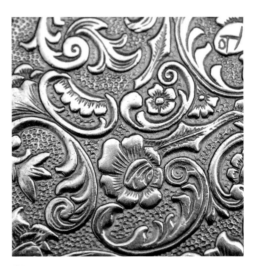

Silver

a summer woman's jewelry

- *Best metals*, either matte or shiny, are platinum, white gold, pewter, or silver.
- *Precious and semi-precious stones* include opal, moonstone, rose quartz, and mother of pearl.
- *Accent stones* include aquamarine, amethyst, pink tourmaline, pink sapphire, pastel blue sapphire, blue topaz, blue zircon, and kunzite.
- *Clear stones* are diamonds, white topaz, moissanite, and cubic zirconia, which are best set in white gold or platinum.
- *Pearls*, whether real or faux, should have a pink or silver overtone.

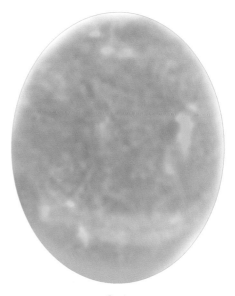

Opal

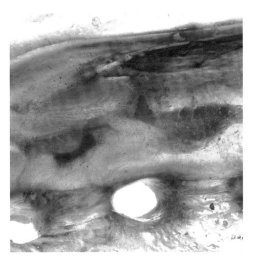

Mother of Pearl

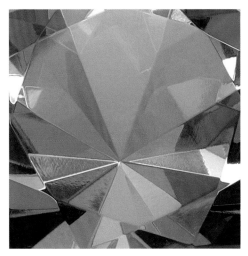

Amethyst

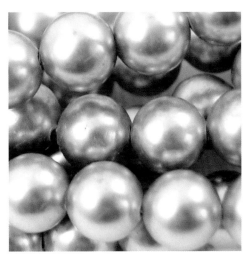

Pink Pearls

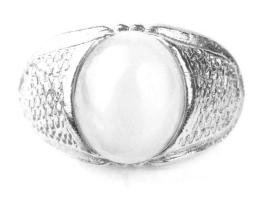

Silver

an autumn woman's jewelry

- *Best metals*, either brushed or shiny, include gold, bronze, and copper.
- *Precious and semi-precious stones* include mandarin garnet, smoky topaz, and green emerald.
- *Accent stones* are tiger's eye, amber, peridot, carnelian, jade, Bahia green tourmaline, fire opal, ruby sunstone, malachite, and jasper.
- *Clear stones* include diamonds, moissanite, white topaz, and cubic zirconia, which are best set in yellow gold.
- *Pearls*, whether real or faux, should have ivory or cream tones.
- *Funky* Autumn looks include exotic wooden jewelry and tortoise shell.

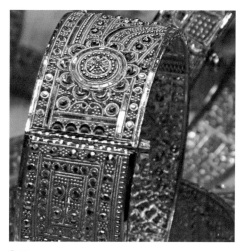

Gold

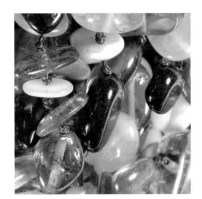

Malachite

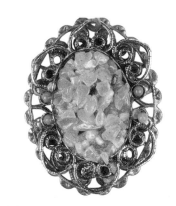

Amber

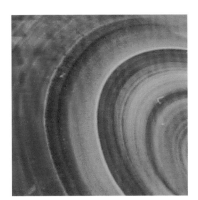

Ivory Pearls

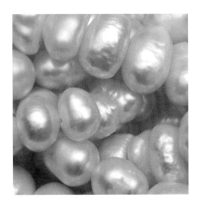

Jade

a spring woman's jewelry

- *Best metals*, either brushed or shiny, are in the gold, bronze, or copper family.
- *Precious and semi-precious stones* include amethyst, Swiss blue topaz, and aquamarine.
- *Accent stones* are coral, jade, citrine, turquoise, peridot, and blue zircon.
- *Clear stones* include diamonds, moissanite, white topaz, and cubic zirconia, which are best set in yellow gold.
- *Pearls*, whether real or faux, should have ivory or cream tones.

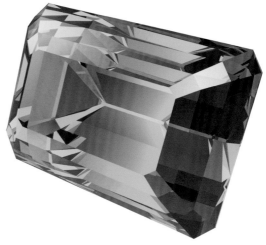

Aquamarine

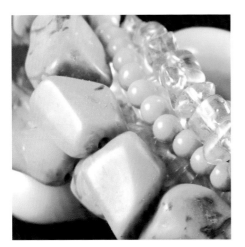

Turquoise

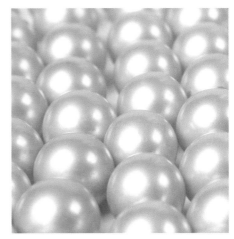

Ivory Pearls

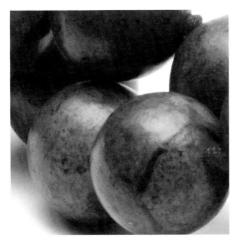

Coral

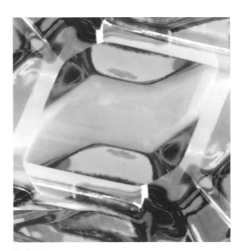

Periodot

Eyeglasses and sunglasses fall under the same set of rules as jewelry because of their proximity to your hair, face, and neck. When choosing eyewear, look for glasses that harmonize with your hair. Follow the silhouette, size, and shape advice of your eye specialists, and pick a frame color from your swatch book. You can expand your eyeglass wardrobe by adding gemstones as accents to the frames. And you can change your sunglass colors to match your outfit, as long as you stay within your seasonal color. If you wear colored contact lenses, make sure that you choose a color that suits your season.

A Winter Woman's Eyewear

Winter women should choose a brushed or shiny silver metal frame. Good colored eyeglass frame options are black, charcoal, navy, red, royal blue, gray, or teal. The best sunglass lens color for Winter women is gray/black.

A Summer Woman's Eyewear

If you'd rather wear a colored eyeglass frame than silver metal ones, then your choices range from light rose brown, gray tortoise, medium gray, gray blue, teal, amethyst, rose, spruce, taupe, light pink, to teal. Sunglasses lens from the blue or gray families suit Summer women best.

An Autumn Woman's Eyewear

Brushed or shiny gold, bronze, or copper metal eyeglasses frames work best for Autumn women. Color selections include deep golden tortoise, golden brown, mahogany, forest green, rust, terra cotta, and olive. The ideal sunglass lens is brown.

A Spring Woman's Eyewear

Colored frames for a Spring woman include golden brown tortoiseshell, turquoise, camel, khaki, and taupe. Do not choose a tone deeper than terra cotta. Spring eyewear also includes shiny or matte gold, bronze, or copper metals. For sunglasses, the ideal lens colors are brown and green.

handbags

No accessory is as indispensable as a handbag. Find a fashionable bag in your color palette that is functional and fits your lifestyle. If a particular shopping season does not offer any bags in your seasonal colors, walk away. You should have a basic leather traditional handbag in your color palette to revert to until more flattering colors are fashionable again. Apply Color Me Beautiful's rules when purchasing nonleather handbags too, whether they be summer straw handbags, fall plaid bags, or satin, jeweled, or silk evening bags. Please note that the days of matching handbag and shoes are gone.

A Winter Woman's Handbag

The Winter woman should carry a traditional leather handbag in black. Her fun fashion choices could be red, pink-to-fuchsia, or Chinese blue. The best evening or metallic handbag for her is in the silver family.

A Summer Woman's Handbag

A Summer woman can choose from gray and navy for her traditional basic leather handbag. When the fashion world selects any light-to-mid-pink or purple for the season, the Summer woman should jump on it! Her best evening or metallic bag is silver.

An Autumn Woman's Handbag

An Autumn woman needs a mid-to-dark brown leather for her traditional leather choice. She should pick her fashion bag from the light-to-dark green or rust or mustard tones. The best evening and metallic bag choices for Autumn women are gold-toned.

A Spring Woman's Handbag

Let's look at the choices available to Spring women. A good traditional leather color choice is in the light-to-medium brown range. When either mid-blue or mid-green bags hit the stores, buy one! Our Spring woman will find many complementary outfits in her closet. In addition, she should choose a gold evening or metallic bag.

shoes

Shoe style choices seem infinite. You can go from casual flip-flops during the day to mink-adorned stilettos at night. Our obsession with shoes is well-fed, but it's all too common to have a closet full of shoes that you simply never wear.

You can tell a lot about a person from her shoes. In the best-dressed woman, shoes complement the total look. That's why it's important to get them right whether you're buying on impulse or out of necessity. Your shoes can match the dominant color of your outfit or the fringe color from an accessory, such as a belt or piece of jewelry. Hosiery should never be any darker than your shoes. Think how easy it will be to go into a large shoe store now. You can just zip past all the shoes that won't match your outfits because they are not included in your color swatch book.

cold weather footwear chart

WINTER	SUMMER	AUTUMN	SPRING
Black	Navy	Brown	Medium
Navy	Gray	Green	brown
Gray	Taupe	Ivory	Ivory
Silver	Silver	Gold	Bronze
			Gold

warm weather footwear

WINTER	SUMMER	AUTUMN	SPRING
Pink	Bone	Bronze	Ivory
Hot blue	Lavender	Green	Bronze
Red	Medium blue	Salmon	Medium
Yellow	Medium pink	Peach	blue
Pewter	Pewter	Gold, bronze	Peach
			Gold

scarves

A scarf in your season can make your out-of-season clothes wearable again. Be sure the scarf matches and blends with the outfit, however. Scarves are one of the least expensive ways to update your wardrobe, especially while you are in the midst of changing into your new color palette. One scarf has ten different uses. It's a cheap and easy way to add sophistication to any outfit. It can alter the appearance of the neckline by filling in a V-neck, covering up a collar, or creating the illusion of a blouse under a suit jacket. Whether your scarf is knotted, twisted, tied, wrapped, or draped, it can alter your current look with a splash of color that reflects today's trends.

Pashmina Shawl

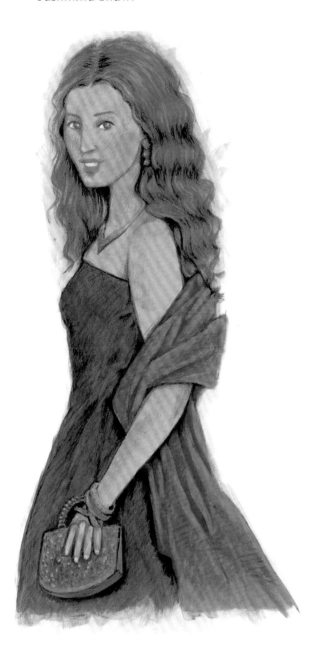

A large Pashmina shawl should be worn off the shoulders and over the upper arm. Loop the shawl behind the body.

The Hacking Knot

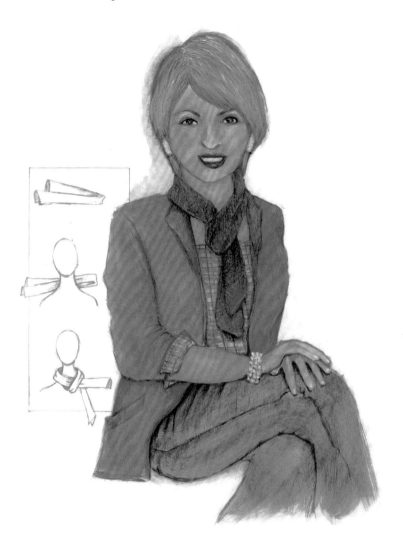

Start with an oblong scarf and fold it in half. Drape the halved scarf around your neck. Pull both ends through the looped end. Tighten, and then adjust. Alternatively, tightly twist the entire length of scarf before you fold it in half. Hold it around your neck with the center loop open. Then pull the free ends through the loop.

Tying a Shawl Wrap

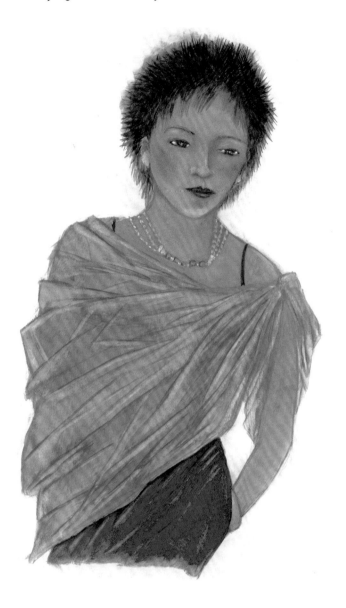

Fold a square scarf that is at least 36 inches square into a triangle. Check that the widest angle falls around the middle of your back. Place around your shoulders, and tie in front. You could also cross over or use a pin to hold it in place. Alternatively, swing the knot to one side and wear it off the shoulders.

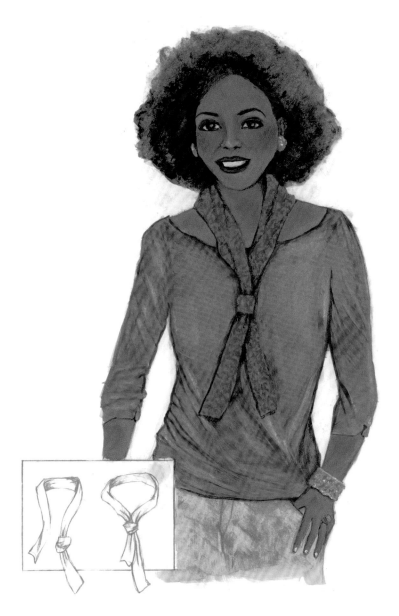

Use an oblong scarf. Tie a loose knot on one end,
and slip the other end through the knot. Adjust tightness.

fur

Fur accessories come in an assortment of choices, such as mufflers, headbands, earmuffs, collars, cuffs, and accent pieces for outerwear. When purchasing real or faux fur, keep *warm* and *cool* characteristics in mind and choose the depth of color based on your season. *Warm* women look best in red fox, whereas a *cool* woman would stop traffic in blue fox. If you want to style it up with something a little funkier, try a pink faux fur neckwarmer if you are *cool* or moss green faux fur earmuffs if you are *warm*.

hats

In the past, a beautiful hat always completed outfits. Today's hats are worn to protect us from the elements. Whether we are wearing a straw hat to shield us from the sun's rays or a cashmere head wrap to ward off the chilly winter winds, we still need to follow our seasonal color rules. As always, be sure to refer to your color swatch book when making a hat purchase.

Your hat color can accent or match your coat, jacket, or top. In the summer months, add a ribbon, scarf, or flower to a straw hat. In the winter, wrap your favorite muffler around your head for protection on blustery days, and wrap it around your neck on milder days. You'll get two different looks from the same accessory.

belts

Today's belts act as another color accent or can be used to complete a monochromatic look. If you are going for a basic look, however, what goes for shoes also goes for belts. If you are *warm*, then basic brown suits you best. Black is the choice for *cool* seasons.

Belts can also mask figure problems. If you have a short waist, buckle a belt over your blouse, sweater, or jacket and below your natural waist line; you will appear to have a longer torso. Beware, however, because the reverse is also true. If you tuck in your top and wear a belt at your waist, your torso will look shorter. Belt fashion trends cycle between the skinny one-quarter-inch type and the five-inch corset type. Keep the classic basic gold or silver chain belt in your wardrobe. Always remember that not everyone can wear every fashion trend, so be content wearing what makes you look and feel your best.

nails

Manicures and pedicures are now more popular than ever. Whether you give one to yourself or go to a nail salon, they are part of your routine. When you select your nail polish color, keep your season in mind. Any color that is in your swatch book will blend with your other seasonal choices.

Cool women should choose a shade in the range of light pink to hot fuschia. A bright red polish with blue tones looks great during the holidays. A silver fleck in the polish or topcoat finishes your *cool* look.

Any shade of coral, salmon, peach, or brown will blend well on a *warm* woman and will match her *warm* clothing. Gold flecks in the polish or topcoat accentuate her *warmth*.

If you want to get a professional manicure but don't wish to make a color statement, get a neutral French manicure.

■   ■   ■

Well-dressed women accessorize. It's an elegant way to raise the bar. Integrate your new palette choices into your wardrobe with new earrings, necklaces, eyewear, handbags, shoes, scarves, and belts. You may be surprised by the sophisticated, polished woman looking back at you in the mirror!

putting
it all
together

Now that you know which of Color Me Beautiful's four seasons categories best describes YOU, the next step is easy. You now possess the knowledge and confidence to recommend to your hairdresser which hair shade is best for you. You can now choose all your foundations, eye shadows, blushes, and lipsticks either from the *warm* or *cool* makeup collection with confidence. Color Me Beautiful's clothing color chart will help you select the outfits that will make you sparkle everyday. And to complete the picture, you can walk into a jewelry store knowing with certainty the recommended range of colors in selecting your necklaces and earrings.

In addition to this book, you may want to use other Color Me Beautiful resources, especially the Web site at www.colormebeautiful.com. There you can find beauty consultants in your area, sign up for a free newsletter, and much more.

about the author

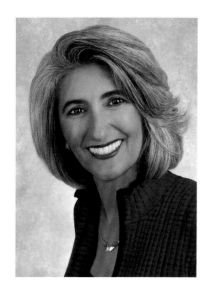

JoAnne Richmond has over twenty years of experience in the image consulting and fashion merchandising fields. She is a graduate of Penn State University with a degree in business. Since 1996 she has been associated with Color Me Beautiful as an Independent Color Consultant. In 2001, JoAnne was selected to become a National Certified Color Analysis Trainer for *Color Me Beautiful*.

JoAnne's experience includes extensive living and traveling throughout Europe, Asia, and the Middle East, where she has promoted the *Color Me Beautiful* concept to expatriate communities. In the United States and abroad, JoAnne educates on color analysis to individuals, to small private groups, and at large conferences. Her goal is promote higher levels of self-esteem and confidence, teach clients to make positive and lasting first impressions, and provide tips on saving time and money.

When not pursuing her Color Me Beautiful career, JoAnne enjoys competitive team tennis, teaching water aerobics, and bible study. She is the proud mother of Scott and Julia, both recent college graduates. JoAnne resides with her husband, Wayne, in Northern Virginia and Florida.

Color Me Beautiful

If you would like to order
your Season's swatch book
in an attractive slim-line wallet, and
your Season's best cosmetic colors,
visit www.ColorMeBeautiful.com
or call 1-800-ColorMe (265-6763)

If you'd like to learn more about
becoming a Color Me Beautiful Consultant,
earning an excellent income
while helping others look their best,
visit www.careersinbeauty.com
or call 1-800-606-3435